The Migraine
Prevention Cookbook

The Migraine Prevention Cookbook

BY JOSIE A. WENTWORTH

Introduction by Katharina Dalton, M.D.

Originally published in England as
The Migraine Guide and Cookbook

DOUBLEDAY & COMPANY, INC.
GARDEN CITY, NEW YORK
1983

Originally published in Great Britain by Sidgwick & Jackson Ltd. as
The Migraine Guide and Cookbook

Library of Congress Cataloging in Publication Data

Wentworth, Josie A.
  The migraine prevention cookbook.

  Bibliography: p. 192.
  Includes index.
  1. Migraine—Diet therapy—Recipes.   I. Title.
RC392.W46   1983   616.8'570654
ISBN: 0-385-18052-7
Library of Congress Catalog Card Number 82–45277

Contents

Items marked with an asterisk may be located by consulting the
Index.

Acknowledgments

I would like especially to thank Katharina Dalton, M.D. (whose idea this book originally was), for her constant support and help in supplying and checking all the medical material, for painstakingly answering many questions, and for her continuing encouragement. My thanks also go to Maggie Black for her contribution to the recipe section and her very valuable help in checking and testing the recipes; to my editor at Doubleday, Louise Gault, for her enthusiasm and encouragement; to my sister, Jill F. Middleton, for inspiring my love of food and contributing many of the recipes; to Carolyn Dehnel for advising on measures, terminology, and availability of ingredients; to Megan Feacham for deciphering my handwriting and typing the original manuscript; to Marcelle Letacq for retyping the recipe section, and to Cedric Marsden for his constant support and help in checking and collating the manuscript.

I am also grateful for the help given me by the following people, companies, and associations: Masa Aoki; Michael Bateman; Wendy M. Clark (Microbiologist, John Harvey & Sons, Ltd., Wine Merchants); Monica Conrady; Jim Dawson; Dr. Edda Hanington (Wellcome Trust); John Holtom; Peter Holtom; Janet Maclean; Jane Pinkerton; Stanley Pauling for his excellent sausage recipes; Dr. Saxby (British Food Manufacturers' Research Association); Carol Hupping Stoner; Maureen W. Wentworth for contributing several recipes; the British Medical Association; the British Migraine Association; Cadbury Schweppes, Ltd., Research Laboratories; *Headache Update* (Organon Pharmaceuticals, New Jersey); Harcourt, Brace & World, Inc.; the Migraine Trust, London; the National Migraine Foundation, Chicago, Illinois; The Office of Health Economics; The Royal Society of Medicine; and *The Journal of the Royal College of General Practitioners.*

Introduction

Migraine is a common and incapacitating disorder that is still listed among the diseases of unknown origin. Much research work is continuing throughout the world; every year more knowledge accumulates and little shafts of light are beginning to appear.

For a migraine attack to occur, certain conditions must first be satisfied. The individual must be susceptible to migraine (it is sometimes difficult to realize there are many lucky folk who have never experienced one). This susceptibility to migraines is usually already present at birth, being frequently inherited through one or other parent, or a grandparent. On the other hand, it may more rarely be acquired as a result of a severe head injury or meningitis. Then there are certain factors that make a susceptible individual more prone to develop attacks, and in this category come tension, stress, fatigue, and lack of sleep. With women there are certain times when they are more liable to develop an attack; these times include the few days before menstruation, the days during menstruation, immediately after childbirth, during the week off the contraceptive pill, and at the menopause. Nevertheless, these factors only increase the tendency to develop a migraine. There still remain those final precipitating factors that trigger a full-blown migraine attack. The best understood of the final trigger factors are the dietary ones. These include going for too long an interval between meals and eating specific foods that the individual's enzyme system cannot dispose of, so that certain substances—vasodilating amines—accumulate in the blood, and open wide the blood vessels of the brain, causing that intolerable throbbing headache.

While none of us can do anything about our parents or our family tree, and it is often hard to ensure freedom from tension, stress, and lack of sleep, nevertheless it is possible to understand and eliminate the dietary factors that can trigger an attack. Today there are many thousands of migraine patients who have successfully mastered the subject and have altered their eating habits so that they can now happily report long intervals between attacks. Indeed, some even speak of their rare attacks as having been "self-induced," adding perhaps: "I couldn't help it—the plane was delayed and no food was available," or "It was such a lovely wedding, how could I say no to the champagne?"

This book fills a vital need in helping migraine sufferers to understand fully the common dietary causes of their attacks and learn how to avoid them. The comprehensive list of appetizing recipes demonstrates that to stick to a migraine diet is no hardship. The recipes avoid the common food precipitants of migraine, but it must be recognized that there are still those few unlucky folk whose attacks are sparked by other foods not considered here. However, for these few the offending food will come to light when several Migraine Attack Forms (see Appendix III) have been completed and studied. These sufferers will need to adjust their diet individually, but having learned the lessons from this book they will find the task of constructing a personalized diet easy enough.

Katharina Dalton, M.D., 1981

Author's Preface

Migraine is one of the oldest known diseases and yet there is still no specific cure. It brings misery to many thousands of people and can be so incapacitating as to disrupt employment and social life. Furthermore, many nonsufferers regard migraine as merely a rather grand name for a headache, so that sufferers are often treated as malingerers and hypochondriacs.

But the pain of migraine is very real indeed and the visual disturbances and constant vomiting or nausea cause much distress to those who experience them. The usual medical treatment consists of strong painkillers and ergotamine derivatives, with rest in a darkened room until the attack subsides. Ergotamine, however, can cause unpleasant side effects when taken frequently or in too high a dosage—not least of these are recurring throbbing headaches! So migraine sufferers often find they are caught up in a vicious circle.

I hope to show in this book that a great deal of self-help can be achieved by every sufferer, principally by strict attention to diet, eliminating certain foods, and eating regularly every three to five hours.

For many years I did not realize that my terrible headaches were in fact migraine attacks. Then one day a friend, who suffered from migraine, saw me during one of my "headaches" and explained to me that I was experiencing a full-blown migraine attack. I visited my local doctor and after much questioning he agreed that I had migraine and prescribed MIGRIL tablets (an ergotamine derivative). These certainly shortened the duration of my attacks considerably, but they did nothing to stop their frequency. And, as you are only allowed to take so many ergotamine tablets in a week, I sometimes found I had to suffer a complete attack without them.

Some time later I consulted Dr. Katharina Dalton, who suggested that I should come off the contraceptive pill. This dramatically reduced the frequency and length of my attacks, but I was still having attacks far too often for comfort, and both my work and social life were being continually disrupted. It was then that Dr. Dalton suggested that certain foods might be precipitating the migraine attacks. It had never occurred to me that I might be allergic to certain foods and I didn't really believe this could be so. I had never noticed any pattern of attacks connected with what I ate. I had long been an ardent follower of the health foods movement and I ate well-balanced, nutritious meals with plenty of fresh fruit and vegetables.

However, I had nothing to lose, so I agreed to keep Migraine Attack Forms (copies in Appendix III), which recorded the foods and beverages I had consumed throughout the 24 hours previous to an attack. They also reported the times I had taken food and drink. It soon became apparent that red wine and cheese were the principal culprits, followed by chocolate and frozen orange juice. Later I added pork and pork products to my personal list of offenders. These had been harder to detect since I found I could eat small amounts with no problem, but if I had pork for several meals or days running, then it appeared to have a cumulative effect.

It was a great blow to find that I was allergic to some of my favorite foods, which previously I had eaten frequently, but I did find that when I excluded them from my diet I could go for long periods without an attack.

Any migraine attacks I have now are usually related to going without food for five hours (daytime) or thirteen hours (overnight) and therefore partially self-induced. I still find it very hard to stick to the strict routine of eating every three to four hours.

Over the years I have learned to cope with my disability and have found that there are still many delicious things to eat that do not include cheese, chocolate, red wine, or citrus fruit—the foods that most often precipitate migraine. In this book I hope to share with you everything that has helped me control my attacks and to give you some idea of the wide variety of dishes for breakfast, lunch, and dinner that can be made without including these foods. I hope, too, that you will experiment for yourself with new dishes and that you will fill in the Attack Forms meticulously so that you can work out your own personal diet plan.

JOSIE A. WENTWORTH

PART I

Migraine—The Facts

1

What Is Migraine?

Roughly half the population rarely or never suffers from headaches, but of the half that does, approximately one in five are migraine sufferers, making the total incidence of migraine sufferers a staggering 8 to 10 percent of the general population.

Many people will ask what is the difference between a headache and migraine? Migraine is a vascular headache that causes intense throbbing pain on one side of the head (either right or left) and is accompanied by nausea, vomiting, biliousness, and/or visual disorders. The sufferer is severely debilitated and cannot continue his or her normal routine. The attacks occur at intervals and ordinary painkiller tablets give little or no relief.

On the other hand, a tension headache is a dull persistent pain often likened to a heavy weight or a tight band around the head. It is not accompanied by nausea and vomiting or visual disorders. The pain is produced by tension and pressure in the muscles of the neck and head, caused by stress and worry. Tension headaches can be chronic and be present more or less continuously, whereas migraine comes and goes in a definite attack. However, it is possible to suffer from both tension headaches *and* migraine.

There are two types of migraine, common and classical. Twice as many people suffer from common migraine as from classical migraine, although sufferers of frequent attacks of common migraine will often have occasional attacks of the classical type.

Common migraine is a unilateral headache accompanied by

nausea and/or vomiting. In classical migraine these symptoms are preceded by warning signs called an "aura." The signs are usually visual and are followed by acute headache pain approximately twenty minutes later. These visual disturbances can be in the form of zigzag lines, colored shapes, or flashing lights. The vision may become blurred and the ability to focus on objects impaired. In some cases, part of the sufferer's field of vision is blotted out completely. In very rare instances, there is temporary paralysis of a limb or even half the body.

Other warning signs include a feeling of extra well-being or a sense of remoteness; sudden excess energy; nausea; extreme hunger or thirst. With these nonvisual warning signs the period between the "aura" and the onset of the headache pain may be much longer than the usual twenty minutes.

What Happens in a Classical Migraine Attack?

Some hours or perhaps only minutes before the onset of an attack, warning signs are experienced. These could include any of the following symptoms:

Visual disturbances: double vision, difficulty in focusing, temporary partial blindness, dazzling colored lights, spots, lines, zigzags, or flashing lights
Numbness, tingling sensation, dizziness, trembling, weakness
Hallucinations
Nausea, vomiting
Sensitivity to noise or light
Depression, irritability, tension
Exaggerated sense of well-being, alterations in mood and outlook
Unusual hunger
Excitability and talkativeness
Speech difficulties
Pains in neck and shoulders
Blotchy patches on skin, or rashes
Inflamed scalp
Unusual pallor, especially in children
Noticeable increase in weight
Swelling of fingers, waist, or breasts

Increase in frequency or volume of urination
Excessive thirst

These signs are all associated with the biochemical changes that occur at the onset of a migraine attack. Latest research indicates that migraine is caused by a malfunction of vaso-active amine metabolism, allowing the release of vaso-dilating amines that cause the blood vessels to dilate or expand. Vaso-active amines affect the size of blood vessels and can cause them either to constrict or to dilate. There are a vast number of different vaso-active amines implicated in the cause of migraine, and these amines are all broken down or metabolized in the body by a group of enzymes called monoamine oxidase enzymes. Research has led us to believe that migraine sufferers have some localized deficiency of monoamine oxidase enzymes, which interferes with their ability to metabolize vaso-active amines.

Migraine, therefore, is a biochemical disorder and changes occur in the affected blood vessels during an attack. It tends to run in families: people are born with a predisposition to migraine, and have a constitutional tendency for their blood vessels to react abnormally to certain stimuli. Vaso-active amines, which are contained in many of the foods we eat every day, can act as a stimulus and cause constriction of large arteries and veins and dilation of smaller arteries and arterioles.

During the first phase of a migraine there is a narrowing of the branches of the carotid blood vessels. This affects the blood vessels on both sides of the head, not just those on the side that will eventually become painful. The retinal vessels on both sides of the head also narrow, and this can be confirmed by examination of the eyes with an ophthalmoscope. In fact, the blood flow in the internal carotid may be reduced to half its previous level.

In the next stage of an attack, the blood vessels on the side of the head where the pain soon develops become enlarged and start to throb. The pain affects primarily the eye and temple, the side of the head, and the back of the neck, but it can spread up from the neck to the top of the head or down into the shoulder of the side affected. The pain is intense and throbs continuously; any slight noise, bright light, or movement, especially when bending down, will aggravate it. Sometimes there are stabbing and shoot-

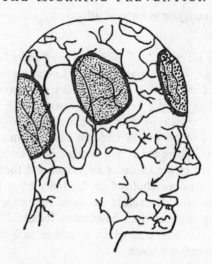

The arteries of the scalp, branches of the external carotid artery.
(The sites of pain in migraine are indicated by the shaded areas.)

ing pains. It is at this stage that the sufferer is forced to lie down in some dark place, with his head buried in a pillow.

During an attack the sufferer looks very pale and ill. He often feels cold and shivery, and has cold hands and feet. In spite of this, his head is very hot. The fact that the blood flow is increased in the painful area could account for the considerable heat given off by the head. It is strange, however, that the face remains white and pale, not flushed, and that the sufferer actually feels cold. The most likely explanation for this is that probably the blood is being pumped to the deeper tissues so that despite the fact that more blood is flowing through the arteries it is not reaching the skin.

The scalp may now be extremely painful to touch and this condition could last for several days after the attack proper is over. The skin is inflamed and the whole area becomes very sore and hot. Sometimes this condition can *precede* an attack.

An attack can last for an hour, several hours, or even several days. Sometimes sufferers have fallen asleep as a result of sheer exhaustion only to find the intolerable pain still there when they awake.

For anyone who has not endured a migraine, it is hard to imagine the agony of an attack. The nearest I can come to an explanation is to ask you to imagine the worst seasickness you have ever experienced and to add to that a throbbing headache that is so bad you cannot move, and you will have some idea of how a sufferer feels during an acute attack.

More women than men suffer from migraine. Figures in a recent survey give a ratio of seven females to four males. The possible reasons for this are discussed in Chapter 9.

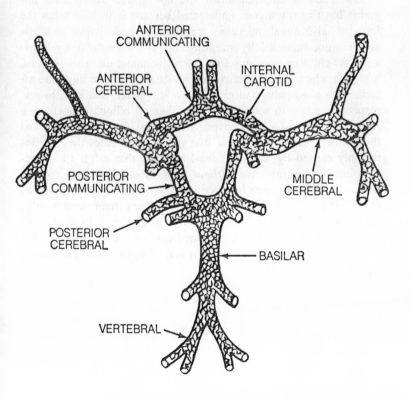

Arteries at the base of the brain, the circle of Willis.

Men suffer more headaches and migraine attacks between the ages of fifteen and fifty-four, after which the incidence tends to decline. Women are not so lucky. They suffer more attacks than men in the age group fifteen to thirty-four, and between the ages of thirty-five to fifty-four attacks increase even more, declining only marginally after the age of fifty-five.

Migraine attacks usually start in the early teens—between thirteen and fourteen. This could be due to hormonal changes taking place, which can be a sensitizing factor affecting amine metabolism. Some women only experience migraine when they have been on the contraceptive pill and here we have very definite evidence of the link between hormone balance and migraine.

Thousands of children under the age of ten suffer from migraine but this often goes undetected because it usually takes the form of abdominal migraine, causing stomach pains and biliousness accompanied by vomiting, but not necessarily by headache. As children have upset stomachs for many different reasons, it is only when the child grows up and starts to have migraine attacks with head pain, nausea, and vomiting, etc., that it is, in retrospect, possible to see that those childhood bilious attacks were really migraine. Recent research shows that many children start their attacks before the age of five and in these cases they are invariably caused by the same food allergies that affect their parents, or by long intervals *without* food. However, where food is involved, the time lapse between ingesting the food and the onset of the attack is much shorter with children than with adults. Therefore mother and daughter could eat the same food and the daughter might start vomiting immediately or within a few hours, while the mother's migraine might not start for twelve to forty-eight hours, or more.

2

Triggers Precipitating Migraine

Although extensive research has already been done and is still continuing, the actual cause of the migraine attack is still not proven. However, research does show that certain things will trigger migraine in susceptible individuals. The list of triggers is extensive, but when these are examined carefully they can be combined within six major categories:

1. Food sensitivity/allergy
2. Hypoglycemia/low blood sugar
3. Tension and stress
4. Water retention
5. Depression
6. Menstruation and the contraceptive pill

It is unfortunate that a large number of sufferers are quite unaware of all the things that can trigger their migraines. For a long time doctors have told their patients that migraine is caused by stress and tension; and so many sufferers have always thought their attacks to be a result of emotional stress, without ever becoming aware of the real culprit.

Even the six categories of triggers, listed above, can be reduced. Tension, stress, and depression can inhibit appetite so that sufferers may not eat; their blood sugar will drop and they will experience hypoglycemic reactions, which they will not recognize as such. In women, water retention is frequently caused by an imbalance of hormones during the menstrual cycle, making the sufferer feel fat and bloated, and often depressed. When a woman feels like this, she does not want to eat. It is very likely that a woman suffering from water retention will lose or restrict her appetite, eat less, and then suffer low blood sugar reactions. And, as every woman knows, menstruation can cause tension and depression as well as water retention and loss of appetite. The Pill can have the same effect, but with the added hazard that it can result in weight gain. A woman putting on weight feels depressed and tries to slim down; she stops eating and consequently suffers from low blood sugar symptoms.

Foods that appear to precipitate migraine are those that contain vaso-active amines. Tyramine, phenylethylamine, histamine, iso-amylamine, octopamine, synephrine, and 5-hydroxytryptamine are just some of the offending amines. However, some people may react to only one or two of these amines while others, fortunately very few, will be sensitive to them all. Some sufferers will not be able to tolerate even a slight trace of any of these amines, while others may be able to cope with them all in small amounts.

To give you an idea of the effect of these amines in susceptible individuals: normally, ingesting 3 mg. of phenylethylamine will induce a migraine; 10 mg. of tyramine will produce a migraine type of reaction; and 100 mg. will cause a severe migraine attack, as will only 8 mg. histamine. As much as 1.5 mg. per gram (42 mg. per ounce) of tyramine has been found in some cheeses.

Recent research suggests that in those with a biochemical defect in amine metabolism, food allergy may be the final precipitating factor in a migraine attack. However, sensitizing factors have usually been present at an earlier stage. Fasting (five hours without food daytime; thirteen hours overnight) may be one such sensitizing factor. Others are the changing levels of menstrual hormones; stress, causing alteration in adrenal hormone levels; lack of sleep, and alteration of body rhythms.

Dr. Katharina Dalton has done much work in migraine research and, in 1975, she conducted a survey on the hormonal aspects of migraine in 2,000 female sufferers. Everyone involved in the survey completed an Attack Form, which, as well as requesting information about the patient's menstrual cycle, asked for a complete list of the foods eaten during the twenty-four hours immediately before the onset of an attack and the time at which the food was eaten. Although this survey had been primarily concerned with hormonal questions, when the Attack Forms were analyzed it was found that 95 percent of the participants had either ingested foods containing vaso-active amines—cheese, chocolate, citrus fruits, and alcohol—or had low blood sugar due to fasting prior to their attack. Fasting was defined as taking no food for five hours in daytime or thirteen hours overnight.

The final question on the Attack Form asked: "What do you think caused this attack?" Only 14 percent mentioned food at all and only 2 percent thought that fasting could have been responsible, whereas stress, worry, and tension were frequently cited. Even when the evidence of food sensitivity was put before the patients, many could not accept it as the cause.

A migraine sufferer myself, I also did not think that food could possibly be the cause of my attacks until I systematically tested each suspect food and completed an Attack Form. The enormous number of severe attacks I experienced during those self-imposed trials did more than convince me that eating what had been my favorite foods had in fact amounted to playing with poison.

The whole question of food allergy and low blood sugar is complicated. We must also consider body rhythms and the individual. No two people are alike, but if you monitor your attacks very carefully you will soon find the triggers that relate to you, and your personal tolerance levels.

Let us look at body rhythms. Throughout the day the body is a hive of activity, keeping everything working correctly, supplying and withdrawing chemicals as and when they are needed. The rhythms of these activities affect our moods, energy levels, susceptibility to illness, and our reactions to food and drugs. Doctors have long known that many drugs are more effective when taken at certain times. You may have noticed that most prescriptions specify when the medication is to be taken: in the morning, last thing at night, before or after food. Armed with this knowledge, let us return to food sensitivity or allergy in connection with migraine. It is possible that you will find you can tolerate a particular food at one time but not at another. I know a number of sufferers who can happily drink orange juice for breakfast but cannot tolerate it in the evening.

Another thing to remember about triggers is that their effect is cumulative. You may be able to cope with one trigger, but add two or three together and it is unlikely that you will escape an attack. For example, a person who has had a stressful day, has skipped lunch, is ravenously hungry, and so decides to eat a bar of chocolate is far more likely to develop a migraine than the same person on a restful day, when he or she has eaten regularly and decides to have a chocolate at the end of an enjoyable meal.

Stress and tension may increase your sensitivity to certain foods. So too do changes in the hormone balance. A woman may find that she can tolerate alcohol for most of the month, but that even one glass on the days in the premenstrual period will induce a migraine. The same could be true of cheese; you might find that as long as you eat small amounts and choose cheeses with low tyramine levels (see Chapter 5), you experience no ill effects. But if you eat cheese when you are upset or worried, or perhaps when you are ovulating or menstruating, the effect will be a severe migraine.

Dr. Dalton has kindly agreed to allow me to quote from some of her case histories[1] to help illustrate the problems involved in spotting migraine triggers. Perhaps you will be able to identify with some of the situations in your own life and see for the first time what actually triggers your attacks.

Time Lapse

CASE 1   A 54-year-old male director suspected that dairy foods provoked attacks and he had successfully avoided them for 3 years, until he was tempted to eat some yoghurt. After 24 hours he phoned to tell me that no dire results had befallen him—but a second call the next day informed me that severe migraine had developed after 36 hours.

It can take anywhere from twelve to forty-eight hours after eating an offending food for a migraine to develop.

[1] Taken, together with Dr. Dalton's comments, from "Migraine—A Personal View," by Katharina Dalton, M.D., *Proceedings of the Royal Society of Medicine,* March 1973, Vol. 66, No. 3, pp. 263–66.

Food Sensitivities

The easiest trigger factors to eliminate are in those patients whose attacks result from tyramine sensitivity, and here one must acknowledge the work of Edda Hanington, who, in 1967, demonstrated the link between migraine and the ingestion of tyramine in susceptible individuals. The commonest food containing tyramine is cheese, but as the time interval between ingestion and onset of attack is usually about twenty to twenty-four hours the cause too often passes unrecognized.

CASE 1   A housewife aged 47 attended with three completed Attack Forms. Together we observed that her migraine had occurred 20 hours after a meal of cheese. Then she suddenly became crestfallen as she recalled that the previous evening she had eaten 4 oz (120 g.) of Cheddar cheese for supper when she was alone in the house. At 4 p.m. that afternoon her husband phoned to say that she was having her worst ever migraine.

Recognition of tyramine sensitivity can alter an individual's life pattern, especially in those whose attacks were previously considered to be of psychological origin.

CASE 2   A financial executive, aged 37, suffered from occasional attacks while working in a London suburb. His firm then moved him to central London and there he had frequent migraine. This was attributed to the extra responsibility entailed in his work. After a year he returned to his former office in the suburbs where the attacks were less severe. It was only when thought was given to the possibility of an offending food that it was appreciated that in central London he often had time for only a quick lunch of a cheese sandwich and beer whereas in the local office there was time for a proper meal. Now he can pinpoint attacks, which are always due to a dietary indiscretion.

Tyramine Sensitivity Diminishes During Pregnancy

CASE 1   A mother aged 34 recognised that attacks were precipitated by chocolate, wine and cheese and was delighted to find that after the first trimester of her second pregnancy she could eat these foods with impunity. As she had planned to limit her family to two she indulged in the best of wines and the most expensive chocolates for the duration of this pregnancy.

Hypoglycemia

There are people whose attacks are precipitated by long intervals without food or preceded by an unprovoked and insatiable hunger. These people are usually referred to as "hypoglycemic" although their fasting blood sugar is usually relatively normal, and insulin-induced hypoglycemia in a diabetic only rarely provokes an attack of migraine. It seems that in these individuals there is a metabolic abnormality with insulin resistance[2] and a defect in breakdown of liver glycogen.[3] Many who claim that attacks are precipitated by fatigue are in this group. They include those who miss a meal when working overtime, the ones who continue gardening until the last glimmer of light has gone, and those who are determined to finish their decorating before stopping for a meal. Attacks among those following a low carbohydrate diet or undertaking religious fasts are precipitated by hypoglycemia. Those who are unable to sleep in at weekends because they wake up with an attack should consider the possibility of hypoglycemia, and try the routine of a late night snack. Hypoglycemia is more common during the days before menstruation and on a postcoital day. The possibility exists that fasting as a cause may be masked by an apparently obvious psychological precipitant (Case 1 below), or by fatigue and tension (Case 2 below).

CASE 1   A housewife aged 42 had a light fish supper on Friday at 7 p.m. On Saturday she rose at 7 a.m., had no breakfast, and went shopping from 8 to 10 a.m. Then a hurried change for her son's wedding, leaving home at 11:30 a.m. Severe migraine with vomiting developed at 2:30 p.m. after 18½ hours without food.

CASE 2   A woman aged 45, mother of three children, part-time clerk. Attacks occurred on Thursday. She attributed the attacks to fatigue and tension, as, after leaving work at midday on Thursday, she would

[2] J. M. Hockaday, D. H. Williamson, and K.G.H.M. Alberti, "Effects of Intravenous Glucose on Some Blood Metabolites & Hormones in Migrainous Subjects," *Background to Migraine,* J. N. Cumings, ed.

[3] J. Pearce, M. A. Ron, and K. L. de Silva, "Further Studies of Carbohydrate Metabolism in Migraine," *Background to Migraine,* J. N. Cumings, ed.

drive 12 miles to her favourite supermarket, buy a week's shopping, then drive home in time to pick up her daughter from school and take her to a weekly dancing lesson. Admittedly it was a tight schedule, accompanied by fear that traffic delays might prevent her completing it, but it was noticed that apart from early morning tea and mid-morning coffee she had no food until 4:30 p.m. The previous evening meal was at 9 p.m., so she went 19 hours without food, taking only drinks.

It is very tempting if you are worried or upset to sit down and have a glass of brandy to calm you down, or a martini to give you a lift. In fact, more often than not, friends and relations will suggest it as instant help. But beware—your body may react to it like poison because it is already working overtime to cope with the stress and it does not have available the chemicals to break down and assimilate the alcohol. Again, if you are working on a very tight schedule and find you have missed lunch, think twice before gobbling that innocent chocolate bar—you could be sticking a knife into yourself!

3

Low Blood Sugar

In the last chapter we discussed migraine triggers and you will perhaps have noticed that all triggers are greatly increased in effect by low blood sugar levels.

The majority of migraine sufferers have a tendency to low blood sugar, which is probably inherited. So what is low blood sugar (hypoglycemia)? It is the opposite of diabetes—the patient produces too much insulin. The exact amount of overproduction of insulin varies enormously from person to person, and although in severe cases hyperinsulin can be fatal, we are now concerned with the majority of cases where the overproduction of insulin as insulin resistance, although way above normal and sufficient to produce some very unpleasant symptoms, is nowhere near danger level.

The symptoms of severe insulin shock are feelings of light-headedness, faintness, palpitations of the heart, and a cold sweat. The person complains of a severe headache and often has double vision. Patients may begin to tremble and become unsteady on their feet. In spite of feeling famished sufferers are likely to vomit any food they have taken to relieve their hunger or, at best, are overcome with waves of nausea. If the blood sugar continues to fall the patient will faint. (Have you noticed how many of these symptoms are the same as those experienced in the "aura" stage preceding a migraine attack?)

Normally, insulin is secreted at frequent intervals in response to the metabolic demand but that is all, whereas the diabetic's secretion of insulin is scanty and insufficient for the body's needs. The hypoglycemic, on the other hand, receives a continuous outpouring of insulin.

Blood sugar is the fuel for every cell in the body. The brain is no exception—it is nourished by the glucose in the blood. So, as blood sugar or glucose levels drop, depression and a state of panic or nervous tension and anxiety result. The brain is literally being starved and is panicking in an attempt to keep itself functioning.

Hypoglycemia cannot be cured or controlled by a miracle drug, but it can be controlled by adherence to a special diet. This places the responsibility for controlling the condition entirely with the patient. This is not easy, as it means sacrificing many of the self-indulgences previously considered relatively harmless.

Before we discuss the diet in greater detail, it is important to understand what happens when food is ingested by a hypoglycemic person. In a hypoglycemic, too much insulin is secreted in response to metabolic demand. The liver uses the insulin and stores too much sugar in the cells, leaving insufficient sugar circulating in the blood. The net result of eating a meal can therefore be a further drop in blood sugar.

You might think that the answer is to add more sugar to your diet. Unfortunately, eating more sugar only aggravates the problem because ingesting it acts as a direct stimulant to the body to produce more insulin and the hypoglycemic is back to square one. Coffee, or rather the caffeine contained in it, is one of many stimulants to the adrenal that indirectly, but nevertheless surely, instigates a chain reaction that ends up with the production of more insulin.

If you are prone to waking up in the morning with a migraine or if you find that a migraine inevitably develops when you have indulged in a Sunday morning lie-in, low blood sugar may be responsible. If the nausea accompanying the migraine is not too severe and you can force yourself to have a hearty breakfast, you may find this is sufficient to disperse the attack. But it is a strong-willed person who can force himself or herself to eat a high protein breakfast without coffee or strong tea, when he or she feels like throwing up. The temptation is to bury one's head in the pillows and try to escape the pain in further sleep. But if you do so, you are likely to be in for a day-long attack.

I have just mentioned the sort of breakfast that should be aimed for; this is indicative of the whole diet that should be adopted if you suspect you suffer from low blood sugar. Incidentally, you need have no fear of adopting such a diet whether your blood sugar is low or normal, for it can do you no harm.

The key to this diet is to eat little and often with high protein and a relatively high fat content (fat helps to depress the activity of the "islands of Langerhans," the glands that produce insulin). Obviously, the fat content should be watched and when you have controlled your condition it should be reduced.

It has been suggested that the action of vaso-active amines is increased if they are ingested with fat. Personally, I try to reduce the amount of animal fats in my diet, and substitute vegetable or sunflower oil whenever possible. Fat can be easily and safely added to the diet in the form of a salad dressing made with a few teaspoonfuls of sunflower oil mixed with a little cider vinegar. Toss your daily salad in this delicious dressing and forget about any other fat. However, if you are on a fat-free diet or have a heart condition, do please consult your doctor before making *any* change in your diet.

The idea is to eat frequent small meals high in protein, low in easily absorbable carbohydrates. Sugar should be excluded wherever possible if not completely, as should caffeine. You should aim to eat a protein snack at least every four hours and to go no longer than twelve hours overnight without food. This diet will not cause an increase in weight because you do not eat *more* food, you simply eat *more frequently.* You will find that protein foods are more satisfying than carbohydrates and therefore you will not want so much.

Low blood sugar sufferers should aim for a diet that gives 80 protein grams per day to start with. Table 1 at the end of this chapter lists protein contents of principal foods. As the blood sugar levels stabilize you may find that you can manage with less protein, but as everyone has a different metabolism you must find your own levels.

A suitable diet for a low blood sugar sufferer would be on the following lines:

On Waking, Before Arising

½ cup pineapple juice

1 cup of decaffeinated coffee (unsweetened, if possible, *or* sweetened with ½ teaspoonful honey)

1 graham cracker

Breakfast

Fresh pear or slice pineapple, or apple or peach or apricot

2 poached eggs on 1 slice whole wheat toast with butter *or* 3 ounces poached or grilled fish plus 1 slice whole wheat bread (a vegetable such as cabbage, cucumber, or celery may be substituted for the whole wheat bread)

Midmorning

¼ cup cottage cheese with 1 graham cracker *or* 1 chicken drumstick

½ cup apple juice *or* herb tea *or* decaffeinated coffee

Lunch

3–4 ounces fish *or* meat *or* 2 eggs (if not eaten for breakfast)

Salad with oil and vinegar dressing *or* small helping vegetables (not too much potato but do not cut out completely unless substituting 1 slice whole wheat bread)

Midafternoon (Tea)

¼ cup cottage cheese plus 1 graham cracker *or* 1 egg *or* 1 tuna sandwich made with ⅓ cup mashed tuna *or* 1 cup milk or milk shake plus 1 whole wheat biscuit *or* ⅓ cup mashed sardines on toast

Dinner

½ cup apple juice

Soup

3–4 ounces fish *or* meat *or* poultry plus vegetables

1 slice whole wheat bread

After Dinner

(Every 2–3 hours before retiring)

½ cup milk *or* ½ cup nuts *or* ½ cup cottage cheese *or* a snack (see Chapter 16).

Obviously this is only a rough guide, to give an idea of what to aim for. Cut down carbohydrates but do *not* cut them out completely. Fresh salads dressed with oil and vinegar (preferably sunflower oil and cider vinegar) can be eaten freely as desired. Out go cakes, cookies, pastries, sugar, sweets, etc., and in exchange eat plenty of fresh fruit. An adequate amount of fresh fruit, salads, and vegetables is important to help you digest the protein.

You may find that after feeling ravenous you can sit down to a high protein meal and, after a few mouthfuls, your appetite suddenly vanishes. This is due to a rapid change in the level of sugar in the blood caused by the activity of digesting the food you are eating. A small spoonful of honey in warm water will make you feel fine in a couple of minutes and you will be able to resume your meal with pleasure. This is also why a candy or small sweet cookie at the end of a large meal can be beneficial to you and help you to have enough blood sugar to digest your meal. But go easy and remember "just a little" is your motto.

Then there is the question of exercise. Exercise quickens the metabolic processes of the body. So if you suffer from low blood sugar, exercise will cause your blood sugar to drop faster than the average person's and increase your need for food.

During my research for this book many people kindly sent me details of peculiarities relating to migraine attacks. One I remember very clearly, since it made headlines in several newspapers, reported that "immoderate sexual indulgence could lead to headaches and migraine"! It went on to tell of a vigorous young man, with a previous history of migraine, who was told by his doctor to slow down his marital transports three days after his wedding because of the migraine headaches they were causing. It further reported that these headaches were often accompanied by tremors and sweating. Various possible reasons were given for these attacks, but I believe the most likely explanation was that the exercise involved in sexual intercourse was causing his blood sugar levels to drop, resulting in headaches, migraine, and other low blood sugar symptoms. So my advice to you is to make sure you have a good meal before any vigorous lovemaking sessions and if they will be going on *all* night incorporate eating as part of your love play, like suggesting a midnight feast of aphrodisiac foods. You will be amazed at your stamina as long as you ensure you have frequent snacks!

Of course this doesn't just apply to sex. A violent game of squash after work will have the same effect as delaying your evening meal by about two hours. I am not advocating that you do not take exercise. Quite the contrary. Exercise is most important for general good health. But it is essential that you realize the effect it has on the metabolism of a low blood sugar sufferer, so that you can adjust your diet accordingly.

Keeping Frequency Charts (see Appendix IV) and Attack Forms to show exactly which days you have migraine attacks and at what time they begin can be invaluable for spotting low blood sugar as a possible cause. Often people do not realize they have been without food for six hours or more unless they have kept a record of when food was taken. Fasting or low blood sugar as a trigger precipitating migraine is far more common than is generally realized. Women seem to be more susceptible to low blood sugar than men and especially so in the days during or after menstruation.

The following case histories are taken from "Migraine in General Practice," by Katharina Dalton, M.D., M.R.C.G.P., and originally appeared in *The Journal of the Royal College of General Practitioners*. They illustrate the way fasting can precipitate migraine attacks.

PATIENT 1   This was a single, 27-year-old female secretary. The attacks were at fortnightly intervals originally on Tuesdays, but later on Thursdays. Further questioning as to what Tuesday activity had transferred to Thursday, revealed that on Tuesday she went direct from work to her hairdresser, having only had a snack lunch. The migraine developed on her way home at about 20.00 hours. When her favourite hairdresser changed her late night to Thursday the patient changed her appointment. Fasting was the trigger factor.

PATIENT 2   This was a male clerk of 42 years, single. The attacks were on weekends and holidays, present on rising 10.00 to 11.00 hours instead of waking with the alarm at 07.30 on working days. These attacks proved to be related to fasting.

PATIENT 3   This was a female medical auxiliary, 54 years old. She rose at 07.30 hours on Saturday, had coffee and a low calorie cracker. She was anxious not to gain weight after having stopped smoking. At 12.45 in a restaurant a severe migraine developed before starting a meal.

PATIENT 4   This was a male sales representative, of 34 years. Sunday

08.00 hours breakfast of porridge, egg and bacon, toast and coffee. He played 18 holes of golf. No further food or drink was taken until 18.00 hours when he developed a classical migraine.

The Sunday morning headache is perhaps the best example of fasting migraine. Often the sufferer has had an early evening meal on Saturday night before going out for an evening's entertainment, perhaps a party or a disco, and then sleeps in on Sunday morning, only to wake with a splitting migraine. The answer to this is to have a late night snack and to put some milk and biscuits by the bed to eat immediately after you wake in the morning. After you have eaten something in the morning, by all means turn over, and go back to sleep.

Sometimes an apparently psychological cause for migraine will mask the real culprit, fasting, as demonstrated in the hypoglycemic cases 1 and 2, described in the previous chapter.

If you think your attack could be due to fasting or low blood sugar, remember that you can easily remedy the situation by eating frequent snacks at three- to four-hour intervals. These snacks can be of nonfattening foods but should be high in protein, and if you divide your total daily calorie allowance into six snacks instead of three meals, this should not affect your weight.

Low blood sugar is something all migraine sufferers should watch very carefully. We know it can precipitate attacks on its *own,* but it can *also* act as a sensitizing factor for food allergies. The following four chapters deal with each of the principal offenders.

TABLE 1
Protein Content of Some Common Foods

The information contained in these tables has been compiled from *The Agricultural Handbook No. 8* and *Home and Garden Bulletin No. 72,* issued by the U.S. Department of Agriculture, Washington, D.C.

When the foods were analyzed they were weighed in grams, so the gram weight in the first column is the exact weight. An approximate familiar measure has been given in the second column for your easy reference. A conversion factor of 28.35 grams to the ounce has been used and then the figure rounded up or down to give an imperial measure. Where practical, a cup measurement is given.

FOOD	WEIGHT IN GRAMS	APPROX. FAMILIAR MEASURE	PROTEIN GRAMS
Bread and Cereals			
Bread			
White, 20 slices	454	1 lb loaf	39
Whole wheat	454	1 lb loaf	48
Whole wheat	23	1 slice	2
Macaroni, cooked	140	1¼ cups	5
Noodles	160	1⅓ cups	7
Oatmeal	236	1¼ cups	5
Oats, rolled	236	3 cups	5
Pancakes, 4 in diam. wheat	108	4 pancakes	7
Rice			
Brown	208	1 cup	15
White	191	Scant 1 cup	14
Spaghetti, with meat sauce	250	Scant 3 cups	13
Wheat germ	104	Scant 1 cup	26
Whole wheat flour	120	1 cup	13
White flour	110	1 cup	12
Dairy Products			
Buttermilk, cultured	246	1 cup	9
Cheese			
Cottage	225	1 cup	38
Cream	28	2 tablespoons	2
Cream, heavy	120	½ cup	2

FOOD	WEIGHT IN GRAMS	APPROX. FAMILIAR MEASURE	PROTEIN GRAMS
Chicken			
Fried	85	3 oz or ½ cup	25
Broiled	85	3 oz or ½ cup	23
Livers, fried	100	3 medium	22
Roast	100	3½ oz or ½ cup	25
Duck, roast	100	3½ oz or ½ cup	16
Lamb			
Braised shoulder	85	3 oz or ½ cup	18
Chop (without bone)	115	4 oz or ½ cup	24
Roast leg	86	3 oz or ½ cup	20
Offal			
Brains, beef	100	3½ oz or ⅓ cup	10
Heart, braised	85	3 oz or ⅓ cup	26
Kidney, braised	100	3½ oz or ½ cup	33
Liver, beef, fried	100	3½ oz or ½ cup	29
Liver, calf's, 1 large slice	100	3½ oz or ½ cup	26
Sweetbreads, calf's, braised	100	3½ oz or ½ cup	32
Turkey, roast	100	3½ oz or ½ cup	27
Veal			
Cutlet, broiled, without bone	85	3 oz or ½ cup	23
Roast	85	3 oz or ½ cup	23
Nuts and Seeds			
Almonds, roasted and salted	70	2½ oz or ⅔ cup	13
Brazils, unsalted, whole	70	2½ oz or ½ cup	10
Cashews, unsalted, whole	70	2½ oz or ⅓ cup	12
Peanut butter			
Commercial	50	1¾ oz or ¼ cup	12
Natural	50	1¾ oz or ¼ cup	13
Peanuts, roasted	50	1¾ oz or ⅓ cup	13
Pecans, whole	50	1¾ oz or ⅓ cup	9
Sesame seeds, raw	50	1¾ oz or ¼ cup	9
Sunflower seeds, raw	50	1¾ oz or ¼ cup	12
Walnuts, raw	50	1¾ oz or ½ cup	7

FOOD	WEIGHT IN GRAMS	APPROX. FAMILIAR MEASURE	PROTEIN GRAMS
Eggs			
Boiled or poached	100	2 eggs	12
Scrambled, omelet or fried	128	2 eggs	13
Yolks only	34	2	6
Milk			
Cow's, skimmed	984	4 cups	36
Cow's, whole	976	4 cups	32
Evaporated, undiluted	252	1 cup	16
Powdered, whole	103	1 cup	27
Yoghurt, of partially skimmed			
milk	250	1 cup	8
Fish			
Cod			
Broiled	100	3½ oz or good ½ cup	28
Fish patties	100	2 small patties	15
Fish sticks	112	5 sticks	19
Haddock, fried	85	3 oz or ½ cup	16
Halibut, broiled	100	3½ oz or good ½ cup	26
Salmon, canned	85	3 oz or ½ cup	17
Sardines, canned	85	3 oz or ½ cup	22
Tuna, canned	85	3 oz or ½ cup	25
Meat, Offal, and Poultry, Cooked			
Beef			
Chuck, pot roast	85	3 oz or ½ cup	23
Corned, canned	85	3 oz or ½ cup	12
Roast	85	3 oz or ½ cup	16
Steak, braising, lean	85	3 oz or ½ cup	24
Steak, sirloin	85	3 oz or ½ cup	20
Stew with vegetables	235	1 cup	15
Beefburger	85	3 oz or ⅓ cup	21

FOOD	WEIGHT IN GRAMS	APPROX. FAMILIAR MEASURE	PROTEIN GRAMS
Soups, Canned			
Chicken or turkey	250	1 cup	4
Consommé	240	1 cup	5
Cream soups	255	1 cup	7
Split pea	250	1 cup	8
Supplementary Foods			
Brewers' yeast, powdered	33	1¼ oz	13
Desiccated liver, defatted	37	1¼ oz	28
Vegetables			
Artichoke, globe	100	1 large	2
Dandelion greens, steamed	180	6¼ oz or ¾ cup	5
Kale, steamed	110	3¾ oz or ½ cup	4
Lentils	200	7 oz or 1 cup	15
Peas			
Fresh or frozen, steamed	100	3½ oz or ½ cup	5
Split, cooked	100	3½ oz or ½ cup	8
Pepper, sweet green, stuffed			
with minced beef	150	5¼ oz	19
Soybeans	200	7 oz or 1 cup	22
Spinach, steamed	100	3½ oz or ½ cup	3

4

Chocolate

Chocolate is the food most commonly suspected by migraine sufferers as the cause of their attacks. Perhaps this is because chocolate is often associated with a treat or pleasure and it tends to be easier to remember when you ate some. A survey of five hundred migraine sufferers who could always relate their attacks to dietary factors showed that 75 percent cited chocolate as the prime precipitant.

Chocolate contains many different amines but, strangely enough, it does not contain tyramine, the amine that first aroused researchers' suspicions and that is found in such large quantities in cheese. It is the amine 2-phenylethylamine that is the prime offender in chocolate. This amine, incidentally, is also found in substantial quantities in some cheeses and wines. It is interesting and useful to note which foods contain which amines because a sufferer may be allergic to one amine and not to another. He or she might be able to eat chocolate with no ill effect, but not cheese.

Bitter and plain chocolate have higher levels of 2-phenylethylamine than milk chocolate and white chocolate. The fermentation and maturation of the cocoa bean greatly increase the amine content and the roasting of the fermented beans causes a seven-fold increase in phenylethylamine concentration. Unfortunately, chocolate just wouldn't taste like chocolate if it was made from unfermented fresh cocoa beans! Fermentation and roasting are essential parts of the processing of cocoa products.

In tests, 3 mg. of 2-phenylethylamine have induced headaches in susceptible individuals. The reaction can vary from person to person; some people may need to ingest far less to get a reaction while others may be able to tolerate a higher level. There is approximately 3 mg. of 2-phenylethylamine in a 2-ounce (60 g.) chocolate bar. Of course this can vary from brand to brand depending on the concentration of cocoa.

As I explained in Chapter 2, there are usually sensitizing factors at work before a trigger food that is ingested causes an attack. The most likely sensitizing factors operating when chocolate is eaten are fasting (low blood sugar) and anxiety or stress. How many of us have been on a shopping spree, not stopped for lunch, and then gobbled a chocolate bar in the car or on the bus home; or have had a rush on at the office so that we skip lunch, feel famished by midafternoon, and so grab a chocolate bar to munch with our afternoon cup of tea? Everyone knows that there is a temptation to eat candies when one is under stress. How many lovers' quarrels or matrimonial upsets are made up with a peace offering of a box of chocolates, and how many of the recipients later develop a migraine, which they automatically blame on the stress caused by the quarrel, never dreaming that it could be the chocolates?

I know of a woman who suffered from premenstrual tension and always became very depressed and tearful a few days before her period. Her husband was very understanding and did everything he could to cheer her up. He made a particular point of bringing her a beautiful box of luxury chocolates at this time each month. She was very touched by his gesture and felt guilty the next day when she had a migraine. It was only when she was being treated for her migraine attacks and started to eliminate suspect foods from her diet that she thought about the chocolates. She asked her husband if he would bring her flowers instead of chocolates for a while. Miraculously her migraines disappeared. Here we have a classic case of hormonal changes acting as a sensitizing factor, causing a stress situation (another sensitizer), and the ingestion of chocolate as the final precipitant of the migraine attack.

Cutting chocolate out of the diet is not easy. There is little else one can substitute for it. The best alternative is the carob pod, also known as the locust bean. It has a chocolate-like flavor and can be used in cooking for flavoring cakes and desserts. It comes from a tree with glossy dark green leaves that grows all over the world. The best variety has a long flat pod, anything from three to twelve inches long, which is dried to make carob powder and other products. The dried pod is brown in color, like chocolate. The chocolate flavor of carob becomes more pronounced when the pod is ground and increases even more when it is cooked.

Although nowadays carob is commonly found in supermarkets it is a health food that has been eaten for thousands of years. It is highly nutritious and is sometimes called St. John's bread because it was believed to have been the food that sustained John the Baptist in the Wilderness.

Unlike cocoa, carob does not have a bitter taste. It contains 46 percent natural sugar while cocoa only has 5.5 percent, so it does not need masses of refined sugar added to make it palatable. In spite of carob's sweetness it contains far fewer calories than chocolate, only 177 calories per 100 g. (about 1 cup) against the 295 calories per 100 g. in chocolate. Carob is in fact an ideal substitute for chocolate for anyone who is dieting. Not only is it much lower in calories, it also contains less than 1 percent fat, while cocoa contains 23.7 percent fat.

Carob can be used in almost all recipes that call for cocoa. However, you may need to use less sugar on account of its natural sweetness. Carob powder creamed with a little milk, then stirred into a glassful of milk, makes a delicious chocolate-flavored drink. A selection of dishes using carob is included in the recipes contained in the second half of this book.

On the candy counter, most confectionery that comes in bars is chocolate-coated even if it is not pure chocolate. It is advisable to stick to nougat, fudge, coconut, or some of the excellent dried fruit and nut bars available in health food stores.

Coffee extract is a good alternative to chocolate for producing sophisticated desserts, and so is butterscotch flavoring. They can be used as substitutes for chocolate in icings, toppings, sauces, and creams.

If you are lucky, you may find you can tolerate small amounts of chocolate provided that there are no other sensitizing factors. For example, a mint chocolate following a meal, when the blood sugar is high, may well be tolerated, but never grab a chocolate bar when you are hungry and your blood sugar is low, or when you feel upset and overwrought. It may well turn out to be the final trigger that tips the scale and induces a migraine attack.

5

Cheese

Cheese is the second of the four main offenders that can precipitate migraine attacks. And how delicious cheese is, the easy nutritious snack, the food that requires no preparation, with its sharp distinctive flavoring for sauces and gratin dishes.

Cheese can be a very difficult food to cut out of your diet. However, as it is the amine content (primarily tyramine) of cheese that can cause migraine and this varies from one type of cheese to another, making some more lethal than others, there may be some cheeses you can tolerate.

It is the same action of tyramine that causes problems for people taking monoamine oxidase inhibitor (MAOI) antidepressant drugs. In fact the reactions experienced by patients on these drugs stimulated research into tyramine allergy and the results have been of great help to migraine sufferers. Therefore, people taking MAOI antidepressants will find some useful tips in these pages.

All the hard, mature cheeses are exceptionally high in tyramine, as are most of the blue cheeses. The tyramine content of cheese can vary from one piece to another of the same type and, of course, different types contain different amounts. The amount of tyramine tends to increase the longer the cheese is matured. Therefore, small amounts of young cheeses *may* be tolerated by some people. Some cheeses contain 2-phenylethylamine and other amines as well as tyramine, so even if the tyramine level is relatively low the level of the other amines may be high, or the combination may increase its toxicity.

In general avoid all hard and mature cheese, sharp cheeses, and the blues. New York State Cheddar is exceptionally high in tyramine and should always be avoided. The semisoft cheeses with the lowest tyramine levels are Munster and Gouda.

Soft cheeses such as Camembert and Brie are relatively young cheeses with lower tyramine content and so may be tolerated in small quantities by some sufferers, especially when eaten at the end of a meal. Cream cheese and cottage cheese have been found to contain *no* tyramine or 2-phenylethylamine or any of the other vaso-active amines, and can therefore be eaten without fear.

In control tests, as little as 6 mg. of tyramine taken orally in food causes changes in the body and produces a rise in blood pressure. Usually 10 mg. of tyramine needs to be ingested to produce a headache, and 100 mg. to cause a severe migraine attack. As much as 48 mg. of tyramine per ounce has been found in some cheeses. Table 2 shows the tyramine content of a selection of common cheeses. However, it must be remembered that this is not the only amine present in cheese. Many cheeses also contain substantial amounts of 2-phenylethylamine and if you are allergic to both amines the cumulative effect can be disastrous. Levels of amines in cheeses can vary enormously from manufacturer to manufacturer. For example, when twenty-five commercial Cheddar cheeses of varying history and manufacturer were tested, the highest concentration of tyramine was as much as 33.99 mg. per ounce and the lowest as little as 0.7 mg. per ounce with an average of 10.88 mg. per ounce. The figures given in the chart are the highest amounts found in the cheeses that were tested, but do remember that the piece of cheese you eat may contain more or less tyramine depending on many factors, such as the manufacturer, how old it is, and how it has been stored. Many cheeses do not appear on the chart because accurate data is not readily available, but that does not mean that they do not contain tyramine or other amines. Migraine sufferers should work on the assumption that all cheeses except cottage and cream cheese contain vaso-active amines.

But remember, migraine is brought about by a cumulation of triggers. Even if you find you can tolerate small amounts of some

TABLE 2
Tyramine Content of Some Cheeses

	mcg. per gm.	mg. per ounce
Liederkranz	1683	48
N.Y. State Cheddar	1416	40
Stilton	466	13
Swiss	434	12
d'Oka	310	9
Blue	266	8
Emmentaler	225	6
Edam	214	6
Romano	197	6
Brick	194	6
Brie	180	5
Process	164	4–5
Munster	110	3
Gouda	95	3
Camembert	86 – 125	2 – 4

The tyramine content is given in micrograms per gram in the first column, which has been collated from authentic scientific data. The second column gives the approximate measure in milligrams per ounce for easy reference. As little as 6 mg. of tyramine can cause a rise in blood pressure, but usually 10 mg. is needed to produce a headache.

cheeses, it would be unwise to eat any cheese (except cottage or cream) when the blood sugar is low—that cheese sandwich at lunchtime or a hurried cheese snack is out. No more cheese and wine parties for migraine sufferers—the combination, especially if you drink red wine, will inevitably result in an attack. Do not eat cheese when under stress or in the premenstruum. Some sufferers may find they have to avoid cheese only on certain days of the month in order to be free of their migraine attacks.

For most sufferers, unfortunately, cheese must be cut out of the diet altogether with the exception of cream or cottage cheese, both of which seem very bland after the rich, sharp flavors of other cheeses. However, they can be livened up. Try adding finely chopped garlic to cream cheese and eating it scooped onto fresh sticks of celery. Cottage cheese mashed into a smooth paste with freshly ground black pepper and chopped olives is a delicious slimming snack. Of course, you can add chopped fruit and nuts to both cottage and cream cheese for an exotic dish. More ideas for using these cheeses in cooking, and substituting them in dishes that normally require a hard cheese, can be found in the recipe section.

It is surprising how many dishes are enriched with cheese, and if the latter is to be omitted from the diet you must be aware of its hidden presence. Mornay sauces always contain cheese; many gratin dishes are topped with cheese; and Parmesan cheese is sprinkled on or included in most traditional Italian pasta dishes. Many cooks include cheese in quiches; scallops in the shell may include a cheese sauce. Traditional French onion soup is served with melted cheese on top, while traditional minestrone soup is made with Parmesan cheese. Out go cheese-flavored crackers and cheesy cocktail nibbles, cheese soufflés and omelets. But on the plus side, almost all cheesecakes are made with cream or cottage cheese, so there is no need to give up these delicious concoctions.

Cheese was first suspected as a possible precipitant of migraine when it was the main food incriminated in the headache reactions occurring in patients on monoamine oxidase inhibitor drugs. In her book *Migraine*, Dr. Edda Hanington tells us:

The way in which the monoamine oxidase enzyme entered the migraine field is interesting. In 1952 a new group of drugs was introduced into the treatment of tuberculosis. These drugs acted as inhibitors of monoamine oxidase enzymes in the body; and it was observed that some of the tuberculosis patients who were treated in this way became noticeably more cheerful. Because of this rise in spirits the drug was tried in patients suffering from depression and a marked improvement in some of them was soon apparent. This led to the introduction of monoamine oxidase inhibitor drugs on a large scale for the treatment of depression.

Despite the fact that thousands of patients in the United States were treated with these drugs no adverse reactions to them were reported for three years. Then reports gradually filtered in of severe headaches associated with a rise in blood pressure which occurred in some of the patients on this therapy.

Careful detective work established that these headaches were associated with the eating of certain foods, notably cheese. The substance contained in the cheese that was responsible for these reactions was found to be tyramine, a name derived from *tiri*, the Greek word for cheese. Tyramine is a vaso-active monoamine.

It is normally broken down in the body by the action of monoamine oxidase and exerts action on blood vessels both directly and through releasing nonadrenaline from its stores.

Although cheese was the main food to be incriminated in headache reactions occurring in patients on monoamine oxidase inhibitor drugs, certain other foods were also found to have similar harmful effects. These foods also were subsequently found to contain vaso-active amines. Owing to the inhibition of monoamine oxidase inhibitor therapy which the patients were receiving, the vaso-active amines in the various foods were not broken down and rendered harmless as they would normally have been and the headache reactions resulted.

The role of monoamine oxidase enzymes in migraine has not yet been determined. It is possible that attacks are associated with a deficiency in part of this enzyme system.

Other foods also found to contain vaso-active amines include: cheese, chocolate, yoghurt, overripe bananas, pickled herring, yeast extracts, and alcoholic beverages—especially Chianti. These foods should be avoided by people on MAOI drugs as well as by migraine sufferers.

6

Citrus Fruits

Citrus fruits, the fruits we are always told are so good for us, come next in the order of offenders in precipitating migraine attacks.

Citrus fruits include the orange, lemon, lime, grapefruit, tangerine, mandarin, and the exotic tangelo fruit.

When citrus fruits were first suspected as migraine precipitants they were analyzed, but the method of analysis failed to confirm the presence of tyramine or octopamine. However, another vasoactive amine was found—synephrine—and a very high concentration of it, as much as 35 mcg. per gram in oranges.

Concentrated fruit juice seems to be the worst offender, especially concentrated frozen orange juice. Possibly this is because the whole orange, including the rind, is crushed to produce the concentrate and there are usually higher levels of amines in the skins of the fruit than in the fruit itself. Perhaps it is fortunate that we do not normally drink the concentrated juice of tangerines or mandarins for they contain far higher levels of synephrine than oranges. Levels of synephrine as high as 125 mg. per liter (2⅛ pints) have been recorded in tangerine juice, and in mandarin juice this can be as much as 280 mg. per liter (2⅛ pints).[1]

I have personally found that a squeeze of lemon or lime juice over a salad or in a cake does no harm and that I can happily

[1] Wheaton and Stewart, *Analytical Biochemistry*.

TABLE 3
Average Content of Synephrine in Citrus Fruit Juices

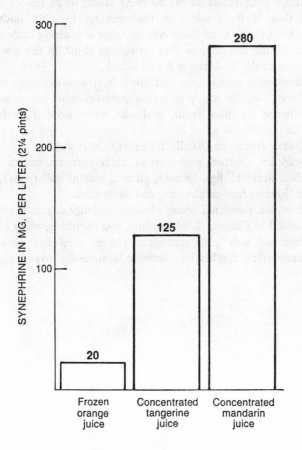

drink tea or soft drinks garnished with a thin slice of lemon. This may be because I never eat the slice of lemon, and the amount of juice that actually permeates the drink is so small that the synephrine content is insignificant. I would not, however, contemplate drinking homemade lemonade, made from crushed whole lemons, sugar, and water or any drink based on real lemon. Artificially lemon-flavored soda drinks are delicious when garnished with a slice of cucumber, a sprig of mint, and lots of ice cubes. Steer clear of frozen concentrated lemon juice altogether.

Fresh orange juice drunk in the morning seems to be less of a precipitant than if it is taken in the evening. Possibly body rhythms account for this, or there may be other sensitizing factors that happen during the day, so that an orange drink in the evening might just be the final trigger for an attack.

As the offender in citrus fruits and juices is synephrine and not tyramine, there may be many migraine sufferers who are completely unaffected by these fruits, and who never need to omit them from their diets.

The following fruits can usually be eaten safely: apples, pears, grapes, pineapples, cherries, gooseberries, black currants, red currants, peaches, apricots, figs, lychees, guavas, melons (all types), strawberries, blueberries, cranberries, and nectarines.

You will notice there are some obvious omissions, and these will be discussed in Chapter 8. Meanwhile, you should be wary of the following, and note your reactions to them carefully: raspberries, loganberries, mulberries, bananas (especially overripe), and plums.

7

And What About Alcohol?

Alcohol is the last of the four major migraine precipitants, and is possibly the most difficult to cut out. When we refer to alcohol we are really thinking about alcoholic drinks that contain at most only 50 percent pure alcohol—the rest of the drink containing many different ingredients to give it a distinctive flavor and color. So we have to consider not only the effect of the alcohol but also the vaso-active amines present in the other ingredients in alcoholic beverages.

Alcohol itself is a vaso-active substance that dilates the blood vessels and increases the flow of blood to the head. Everyone knows the flushed face of someone who has had too much to drink at a party, or the ruddy complexion of a drunkard. If enough alcohol is imbibed it will give anyone a very bad headache and a nasty hangover, regardless of whether he or she is a migraine sufferer or not. However, tests have shown that the severity of the headache and hangover depends more on the type of drink that has been consumed than the actual alcohol content. If you drink alcohol alone you can tolerate far more with no ill effects than if you drink it mixed with other flavoring and additives. It is interesting to see that the alcoholic drinks that contain the highest levels of vaso-active amines are the same drinks that will produce the worst hangovers for any drinker.

The actual pure alcohol content of drinks normally available in bars and liquor stores is relatively small, usually between 50 and

60 percent. Spirits average about 40 to 50 percent; fortified wines (ports, sherries, vermouth, etc.,) 17 to 23 percent; wines 11 to 12 percent; and beers often as little as 6 to 7 percent.

So what to drink and when to drink? It is wise to restrict your drinking habits so that you drink long drinks rather than short ones. Remembering that migraine triggers are cumulative, do not drink alcohol when you are hungry and your blood sugar is low. Beware of cheese snacks and nibbles; cheese and wine parties are out for a migraine sufferer. You may be able to stand one without the other but there is not much chance that you will be able to consume them together without getting a migraine as a result. As cheese is so frequently served with alcoholic drinks, it is worth remembering that this can be a lethal combination.

For many years I suffered regular migraine attacks on Saturday evenings or Sunday mornings. They caused much misery and played havoc with my social life. All sorts of reasons were suggested for these attacks, including one that really annoyed me; it was intimated that obviously I didn't like weekends and was using my migraine attacks as an excuse for not going out! When I started to keep migraine Attack Forms the reason for my attacks stood out so plainly I could have kicked myself. It had become a habit of my husband's and myself to sleep in on Saturday morning, and then do the week's shopping together, ending up at our local wine bar where we often met friends for lunch. Invariably our meal consisted of a bottle or two of wine (usually red, our preference) and a large helping of bread and cheese—usually Brie or Cheddar—followed by coffee. By switching to dry white wine and cold beef or a 100 percent beef hamburger and salad I was able to eliminate these migraine attacks completely.

Alcohol is a food similar to sugar in that it provides the body with calories (energy) but none of the other nutriments essential to health. It is absorbed into the bloodstream as soon as it comes into contact with the walls of the stomach. Alcohol is absorbed more slowly when the stomach is full, so try to restrict drinking to mealtimes, or at least try to eat something when you are drinking, or before going out for a drink.

Alcoholic drinks are normally divided up into spirits, wines, cocktails, and beers and we will look at them under these groups.

Spirits

A migraine sufferer should try to avoid spirits whenever possible because of their high alcohol content. However, if you must drink spirits go for gin or vodka and avoid brandy, whiskey, and Bourbon. Brandy is worse than whiskey or Bourbon. The better the brandy (the longer it has matured in the cask), the bigger the hangover and migraine attack. Orange is a favorite accompaniment to both gin and vodka but for amine-sensitive people drinking this combination is asking for trouble. You may be able to get away with a few gins but adding orange to them may just tip the balance and cause a full-scale migraine. For the same reason beware of liqueurs made with oranges, such as Grand Marnier, orange curaçao, or Cointreau. In fact, all liqueurs should be thought about very carefully.

Wines (table wines and fortified wines)

Vaso-active amines that have been found in significant quantities in wines are: tyramine, phenylethylamine, and histamine. Fortunately, the amine content varies considerably, depending on the type of wine that you drink. One survey of the histamine content shows a variation of as much as 0 to 30 mg. per liter (2⅛ pints).[1] The level reported to induce headaches in susceptible persons was found to be 8 mg. per liter (2⅛ pints). Histamine is present in larger quantities in red wine than in white wine.

Vaso-active amines are products of bacterial fermentation and are therefore found in larger quantities in young rather than more mature wines. So a young California red wine, for example, is not for migraine sufferers.

Phenylethylamine has been found in port and Madeira wine, so it is reasonable to suppose it is also present in other red table and fortified wines such as red vermouth. Red wines generally contain higher levels of vaso-active amines than white wines; this is especially so as regards tyramine. As much as 25 mg. per liter (2⅛ pints) of tyramine has been found in Chianti. As you need

[1] C. S. Cugh, "Measurement of Histamine in California Wines," *Journal of Agricultural Food Chemistry.*

only about 10 mg. tyramine to induce a migraine, half a bottle of Chianti could give you a very severe attack.

Red wines are made from the fruit pulp and crushed skins of black grapes, which contain high levels of amines, while rosé and white wines use only the fruit pulp without the skins. Studies indicate that wines that have been heated during their preparation contain even higher levels of amines. This would account for the higher levels found in red wines and ports, since these are often heated to extract more color from the grape skins.

A certain amount of red wine is often added to sweet sherries to give them a greater depth of color, and this coloring wine has also been heated. This could explain why some people cannot tolerate sweet sherry, but can manage a little dry sherry. However, recent research shows that *all* sherries, sweet and dry, contain high levels of vaso-active amines of many different types, and should generally be avoided by migraine sufferers. It is also worth noting that the amines in sherry become more active when heated, so that when used in cooking, sherry can become a very potent migraine precipitant, particularly in flambé dishes.

Dry white vermouths and white martinis are relatively safe to drink. With regard to other drinks, I suggest that you try them out to find out what suits you. But remember to avoid sherry and all those drinks based on red wines and brandy.

So let us sum up the position regarding wine. Red wines contain higher levels of amines than white wines, so it would be wise to avoid all red wines, especially Chianti. A light dry white wine would probably be tolerated by most people and I suggest a Riesling or Pinot Blanc. Remember, young wines have a higher amine content, so choose a mature wine. Cheap wines contain more impurities, so it is worth paying for a better quality wine, and anyway you can afford to pay more if you are going to drink less of it!

If you are buying French wines, choose those with the *appellation d'origine contrôlée label*. If you are buying German wines, choose a *Qualitätswein bestimmten Anbaugebiet* (Q.b.A.), which is a quality wine from a named area. Preferably, try to buy *Qualitätswein mit Prädikät* (Q.m.P.), which is a natural quality wine with special attributes, made without sugar. If you are buying California wines, go for a good Sonoma or Napa Valley white.

To make your drinking time longer, try mixing an equal amount of dry white wine with carbonated water, and adding ice for a long cool drink. Dry white wine mixed with apple juice and chilled is also a most refreshing drink.

There is no data available regarding homemade wines, and it would be very difficult to test these, as they are not made under controlled conditions. As a general rule, I would avoid home-made wines made from roots or leaves, and stick to the fruit- or flower-based wines that produce white wine. I would avoid any-thing that produces a strong sweet red wine, but I would venture to try a wine that is light and white, and dry, not sweet.

Cocktails

I think the easiest thing to do with cocktails is to list the most common with their usual ingredients. Those cocktails that are marked with a dagger are the ones that should be avoided.

Bacardi Cocktail† 2 parts Bacardi rum, 1 part fresh lime juice, 1 part grenadine

Bloody Mary Vodka and tomato juice with Worcestershire sauce

Brandy Sour† 1 part lemon juice, 3 parts brandy, ½ teaspoon fine sugar

Bronx† 1 part dry gin, 2 parts orange juice, 2 slices fresh pine-apple

Bucks Fizz† Champagne with fresh orange juice

Champagne Cocktail† Champagne with brandy, sugar, and dash of angostura bitters

Chicago† 1 jigger brandy, dash of curaçao, dash of angostura bitters, top up with iced champagne

Gibson Girl ½ French vermouth, ½ dry gin

Gimlet ½ dry gin, ½ lime juice cordial

Gin Fizz† Gin and fresh lemon juice

Gin Sling† 3 parts dry gin, ½ part cherry brandy, ½ part lemon juice, 1 teaspoon sugar, piece of lemon peel, dash of angostura bitters

John Collins† 1 part fresh lemon juice, 3 parts dry gin, 1 teaspoon fine sugar

Manhattan† 1 part dry vermouth, 1 part sweet vermouth, 2 parts Bourbon whiskey, dash of angostura bitters

Martini Large measure dry gin, dash dry vermouth, olive

Negroni† 2 parts dry gin, 1 part sweet vermouth, 1 part Campari with twist of orange

Scarlett O'Hara† 1½ jiggers Southern Comfort, 1½ jiggers cranberry juice, juice of ¼ lime

Snowball ⅙ crème de violette, ⅙ white crème de menthe, ⅙ anisette, ⅙ fresh cream, ⅓ dry gin

Stinger† 1 part white crème de menthe, 2 parts brandy

Whiskey Sour† 1 part lemon juice, 3 parts whiskey, ½ teaspoon fine sugar, dash of angostura bitters

White Lady† 2 parts dry gin, 1 part lemon juice, 1 part Cointreau, teaspoon egg white

Beers

Beers do contain vaso-active amines but in relatively small amounts. The tyramine content has been found to be 2 to 4 mg. per liter (2⅛ pints); as 10 mg. tyramine will usually induce a migraine, you would have to drink at least 2½ liters (5⅜ pints) of beer to precipitate an attack. However, there are other amines in beers and the cumulative effect of all the amines plus the alcohol content itself could tip the balance on a much lower consumption. So I would say you are fairly safe with beers, but watch out they don't catch you unawares. I know one lady who enjoyed a regular bottle or two and suffered no ill effects at all except during the premenstrual period, when a bottle would precipitate a migraine attack.

There are many drinks I have not included because I have no data to indicate whether they are good or bad for you. I suggest that if you enjoy them, you should drink them until your Attack Form proves otherwise!

8
Other Offenders

You have carefully excluded the four main precipitants of migraine: cheese, chocolate, citrus fruits, and alcohol. You are on a high protein diet, and are eating regular meals/snacks every three to five hours, thereby eliminating the possibility of low blood sugar, but you are still getting the occasional unexplained migraine.

There are other foods that contain tyramine, phenylethylamine, and additional vaso-active amines that I have not mentioned in previous chapters because they are foods that you may eat only occasionally. There are also a number of foods that we know cause allergic reactions (not only migraine attacks, but rashes, nausea, vomiting, or stomachaches) in many people who do not necessarily suffer from migraine. We are not sure what the substance in these foods is that causes the allergic reaction, but we do know that in a migraine sufferer such a reaction can take the form of a full-blown migraine attack.

There are also foods that under normal circumstances have insignificant levels of vaso-active amines, but occasionally—perhaps due to growing or storing conditions—the levels may become unusually high and can result in an allergic reaction in a migraine sufferer. Whenever a sufferer has complained of an acute reaction to a food that would not normally be high in these amines, and it has been possible to analyze the offending food, the latter has always been found to have unusually high vaso-active amine levels.

After cheese, chocolate, citrus fruits, and alcohol, the next most likely culprit in precipitating a migraine attack is pork. In fact, some migraine sufferers have found that pork is the only food they cannot tolerate. Pork, of course, includes all pork products: ham, bacon, sausages (even those marked "beef" often also contain pork—so read the labels carefully), pâté, pastes, and liver sausage that contain pork meat, fat, or liver, frankfurters, hot dogs, pork-based salamis, cold meats, and meat loaves. Pork or ham is used to flavor so many dishes that all labels should be scrutinized to see if the product contains pork. Pea and bean soups often include ham pieces, as do many chicken and turkey pies. Terrines and pâtés, even if they do not include pork meat or liver, are often wrapped in bacon.

It is worth remembering that the longer a product has taken to mature, the higher the vaso-active amine content is likely to be.

Some sufferers may find they have to avoid pork and pork products altogether; others, like myself, may be able to tolerate small amounts. But beware of the cumulative effects and try not to have pork or ham three meals running, or on several days in succession. Give your body a chance to metabolize the difficult food before giving it another dose to deal with!

The following foods are relatively high in the offending amines, but it is not likely they will occur regularly in your daily diet and therefore your reaction to them may not be immediately apparent.

Normally 10 mg. tyramine is required to induce migraine, though it can be very much less.

Raspberries

Very high in tyramine. They have fifteen to twenty parts per million. About 8 ounces are usually enough to precipitate an attack, but many people have reported that far less affects them.

Avocados

Tyramine content is 6.5 mg. per ounce, but they also contain other vaso-active amines: serotonin, 3 mg. per ounce, and dopamine, 1 to 1.5 mg. per ounce. An average avocado would weigh 9 ounces (250 g.), which could contain as much as 99 mg. of vaso-active amines. Normally only half is eaten at a time but this could still account for a substantial intake of these amines.

Yeast Extracts

Yeast itself does not contain tyramine, but the preparation of yeast extract by autolysis and the subsequent fermentation leads to tyramine formation. Commercial yeast extracts can contain 42.5 mg. per ounce tyramine and 57 mg. per ounce histamine, which is as high as some cheeses. Also, don't forget amines are absorbed better in fat, so bread and butter and a savory yeast extract would be more easily absorbed than bread and yeast extract alone.

Pickled Herring

The presence of tyramine in this food can be as high as 85 mg. per ounce.

Often the skin or peel of a fruit or vegetable is exceptionally high in amines, while the pulp or flesh has relatively insignificant levels. We have already mentioned this with regard to oranges in Chapter 6 and I now want to draw your attention to other foods where eating the skin or peel can be hazardous, though you are less likely to get a reaction from eating the flesh alone.

Bananas

The level of tyramine increases as bananas ripen and is very high in overripe ones. Banana skin is very high in amines, and the fruit contains 2 mg. per ounce tyramine, 8 mg. per ounce serotonin, and 2 mg. per ounce dopamine. Migraine sufferers should eat only fresh, medium-ripe bananas.

Beans

Normally, these produce a reaction only when the pod, which contains dopamine, is eaten at the same time, but all beans should be eaten cautiously.

The following list includes foods that contain vaso-active amines, but not normally at significant levels. However, sufferers have reported reactions to these foods in some instances so I list them in case you should also react to them.

Tomatoes

Usually only when you are consuming a large amount of concentrated purée or juice.

Onions

Especially when fried, but also when eaten raw in salads or as a garnish. Onions, however, can be rendered harmless if they are blanched before they are eaten. This is done by putting them into cold water, bringing them quickly to the boil, then throwing away the water and using the onions as usual.

Commercial Malted Milk Beverages

Contain amounts of tyramine similar to those contained in oranges and onions.

Red Plums

Can be offenders if eaten in any quantity. Yellow plums do not seem to have the same effect.

Eggplant

This vegetable is usually cooked and eaten in its skin. It may be less of a problem if it is peeled, as amines appear to concentrate in the skins of fruit and vegetables.

Monosodium Glutamate

Used for flavoring in many convenience foods and in Chinese dishes. Because many people experience allergic reactions to MSG, its use in Chinese food has given rise to what is known as the Chinese Restaurant Syndrome.

White Sugar

I personally found a great reduction in the frequency of my attacks when I switched from white sugar to honey for sweetening.

Coffee

I have already discussed the effect of caffeine on low blood sugar in Chapter 3. However, it is amazing how many migraine sufferers drink large quantities of strong "real" coffee every day. I recommend changing to a decaffeinated variety if possible, or a "mild" instant variety. Some people, however, cannot drink instant coffee at all. This is usually because powdered barley is added to many instant coffees, including the decaffeinated variety. It is the barley, which contains gluten, that is causing the problem rather than the coffee.

Shellfish

Prawns, shrimps, crab, lobster, mussels, cockles, clams, and oysters should all be eaten with care, for many people are allergic to some or all of them.

Gluten

There are a few people who have problems with the gluten in flour. These sufferers tend to have their headaches at absolutely regular intervals every ten to twelve days, without exception, holiday, no holiday, Sundays or weekdays. Such people often have a history of food fads and problems in childhood, which gradually develop into migraine attacks in adult life.

Some migraine sufferers say that they react to milk, cream, and butter, but there is no real evidence to show why this should be so. I venture to suggest that the cause of the attack may be low blood sugar rather than the food consumed.

I cannot emphasize enough that migraine is almost always caused by cumulative triggers and an accumulation of amines in the system that are not metabolized so that, when they reach a critical level, their vaso-activity precipitates a migraine attack.

9

Hormones and Migraine

This is a chapter primarily for women. While it seems unlikely that hormone changes alone can precipitate migraine, they definitely can affect the body's tolerance of specific foods. It may be that you can happily eat all foods throughout the month with the exception of four or five specific days.

Research[1] has shown that female migraine sufferers (whether or not they have pronounced menstrually related migraine) have similar hormone levels, and these levels are different from those found in women who do not suffer from migraine.

Migraine sufferers were found to have significantly higher levels of mean plasma estrogen throughout most of their menstrual cycle, but particularly low levels of progesterone in the late luteal phase when there should normally be a high level. Some studies have found that their levels of mean plasma prolactin, however, were lower than normal throughout the cycle. Experimentally, it has been found that ovarian steroids influence prolactin release and the hypothalamic serotoninergic and dopaminergic mechanisms are also involved. Further research may be able to link these hormonal differences to abnormality in the hypothalamic neurotransmitter mechanisms. This is of special interest as we

[1] M. T. Epstein, J. M. Hockaday, and T. D. R. Hockaday, "Migraine and Reproductive Hormones Throughout the Menstrual Cycle," *The Lancet*.

know that migraine sufferers have difficulty metabolizing serotonin and other amines.

While some women suffer only from menstrually related migraine and so know exactly which days they will have attacks, many women suffer from migraine at other times as well, but are still particularly prone to attacks at certain times in the menstrual cycle.

The changing levels of menstrual hormones appear to be a significant sensitizing factor. It is interesting to discover that women taking the estrogen/progestogen contraceptive pill are particularly sensitive to cheese (48 percent) and alcohol (28 percent) precipitating attacks. The incidence of migraine on Day 14 is especially high in this group also. Women who have had a hysterectomy, on the other hand, tend to be more sensitive to fasting (91 percent) and eating chocolate (47 percent) as migraine triggers (see Table 4).

Women who suffer from menstrually related migraine tend to be those who also suffer from the premenstrual syndrome, with symptoms such as tension, fluid retention (and associated weight gain), breast discomfort, and swollen ankles, etc. In fact, it is unusual to have menstrually related migraine without these other symptoms.

The migraine attacks of these women probably commence with the onset of menstruation and they can expect relief from attacks during middle and late pregnancy. Research by the Radcliffe Infirmary, Oxford, England, shows that 80 percent of women sufferers found their migraine completely disappeared during pregnancy after the second missed menstruation, and 60 percent found significant relief. Unfortunately, there appears to be no significant permanent change or improvement until the menopause.

It would seem that pregnancy is the time to indulge oneself in all those delicious chocolates, French cheeses, oranges, and grapefruit.

The worst days of the month for migraine attacks are days one to four of the menstrual cycle, when 29 percent of all attacks occur. (Expected incidence if attacks were evenly distributed throughout the cycle would be 14 percent.) There is a significant increase in sensitivity to all dietary factors in attacks at this time: 31 percent affected by fasting; 30 percent by citrus fruits; 29 per-

TABLE 4
Dietary Factors present in Women under 45 years in relation to the Contraceptive Pill and Hysterectomy

	NUMBER OF ATTACKS	CHOCOLATE	CHEESE	CITRUS FRUITS	ALCOHOL	FASTING
		%	%	%	%	%
Takers	262	35	48	20	28	75
Ex-takers	344	33	44	16	26	73
Nontakers	488	41	34	18	23	61
Hysterectomy	55	47	29	25	18	91
Probability		< 2.5%	< 0.1%			< 0.1%

< = less than

cent by cheese; 28 percent by chocolate; and 27 percent by alcohol. See Table 5.[2]

Other possibly sensitive days, of less significance but still worth watching, are those in mid-cycle (when ovulation occurs) and the days immediately preceding and following the period.

As everyone is different, every menstrual cycle is also slightly different. The woman whose period lasts eight days will have hormone changes at slightly different times in the cycle from the woman whose period lasts only four days.

While the final precipitating factor triggering a migraine attack is fasting or ingestion of specific food, there are obviously many sensitizing factors that may be present at an earlier stage. For example, stress causes alteration in adrenal hormone levels, and lack of sleep or alteration of the diurnal rhythm affects the hypothalamus, which in turn can affect ovarian hormones.

Many women find that they first experience severe migraine when they go on the estrogen/progestogen contraceptive pill. There are many reasons why this should be, but it is obviously related to an upset in hormonal balance.

We know that women with a shortage of progesterone are those most likely to develop menstrually related migraine. However, it is unfortunate that the man-made progestogen contained in the Pill is *not* the same as the pure progesterone produced by the ovaries (which is not assimilable by mouth). Progestogen is a synthetic substitute that actually lowers the blood progesterone levels, and so makes matters worse. So changing pills to different estrogen/progestogen combinations will not help at all, and these women would be well advised to try some other means of contraception.

However, without getting drawn too much into the complexities of the Pill, it may be possible to avoid Pill-induced migraines simply by eliminating the foods that I have listed in previous chapters and avoiding low blood sugar situations.

[2] Katharina Dalton, M.D., *Study of 2313 Spontaneous Migraine Attacks,* February 1975.

TABLE 5
Dietary Factors present in the Menstrual Cycle

DAY OF CYCLE	1 – 4	5 – 8	9 – 12	13 – 15	17 – 20	21 – 24	25 – 28	TOTAL ATTACKS
Chocolate	28*	11	10	16	12	8	5	326
Cheese	29*	14	9	16	11	7	14	349
Citrus Fruits	30*	13	10	11	11	7	17	169
Alcohol	27*	14	9	14	11	7	18	249
Fasting	31*	14	10	12	10	9	14	596

* = Probability exceeds 0.1%

[Tables 4 and 5 taken from *Study of 2313 Spontaneous Migraine Attacks*, Katharina Dalton, M.D., February 1975.]

10

General Self-Help

Get Yourself Right

There is nothing so debilitating as severe pain, and anyone who suffers from migraine will tell you of the utter physical and mental exhaustion that follows a severe migraine attack. Obviously, the body has had a lot to cope with and anyone suffering frequent attacks is bound to find his or her general health is affected.

The body is using all its reserves to cope with attacks, so there may be a sort of general fatigue at other times. Luckily, the body has marvelous recuperative powers if only we give it the right treatment—and that, of course, means attention to diet, coupled with a calm mind.

A few simple changes can make an enormous difference. Try to eat 100 percent whole wheat or whole grain bread. It may taste a little strong to begin with, but you will acquire the taste and I'm sure after a few weeks you will not want to eat processed white bread. You will also find it is more filling and satisfying than its white counterpart so that one or two slices will be all you want to eat at one time. However, the phyton contained in whole wheat bread prevents absorption of calcium so you must make certain that calcium deficiency does not result from this change—particularly if you have already been advised to stop eating cheese and drinking milk. Make sure your diet includes plenty of fresh fruit and vegetables and that some of the vegetables are eaten raw in the form of salad every day. Vegetables are most delicious and nutritious when cooked lightly and quickly. We can learn a lot from the Chinese about how to cook vegetables to retain all their crunchiness and goodness.

Regular meals are particularly important for migraine sufferers —little and often is the rule. In fact many doctors and nutritionists believe that this is best for everyone! Reduce your alcohol consumption—water down drinks with carbonated water, ginger ale, or lemonade, etc.—and always try to drink on a full stomach and not before 6 P.M. Go easy on coffee, too (real and instant), and try to drink decaffeinated instead.

When under stress or overwrought, take a small spoonful of honey to help you raise your blood sugar enough to digest whatever food you eat. Some people also find a couple of spoonfuls of cider vinegar mixed with a little water is a great help to a nervous digestion.

I have found it very beneficial to cut out white sugar. If you have a very sweet tooth, you may throw up your arms in horror at this suggestion, but in fact it is not so difficult. Try using honey for sweetening—it is, in fact, much sweeter than sugar, so you will need to use less and once you have become used to its flavor you will find it is very pleasant in tea and coffee and fruit puddings, pies, and cakes.

Once you have established yourself on a healthy, nutritious diet, make sure you incorporate some exercise in your daily life— nothing violent, at least not to start with, and remember the effect exercise has on metabolism and blood sugar. So the rule is gentle exercise, walking, jogging, dancing, or swimming, and yoga.

Yoga can have many benefits. It is a very gentle form of exercise where the individual can gradually build up his or her strength and increase the amount of exercise as and when able to do so without straining the body. It is particularly good for those people who have not taken any exercise for a few years. Do not be put off by those complicated postures; you are not expected to be able to do them straightaway, and many people who have practiced yoga for years will not be able to do them. That does not mean they are not deriving enormous benefits from the exercises and postures they *can* achieve. The second and almost more important benefit of yoga is that it teaches relaxation—a condition most migraine sufferers find hard to achieve and yet it is especially good for them.

Howard Kent, of Yoga for Health Clubs, has worked with many migraine sufferers in England and he believes that a lot of the pain of migraine can be relieved by a controlled program using yoga techniques. I am sure that anyone who cares to take up yoga will find it extremely beneficial and helpful not only for their migraine but for their general health and well-being.

There are also an increasing number of relaxation classes being held throughout the country; and relaxation cassettes can also be purchased to enable people to learn to relax at home.

What You Can Do to Help Yourself in an Attack of Migraine

The earlier in an attack that you take action, the more likely you are to be able to reduce the pain and length of the attack. First and foremost, try not to panic and become tense in anticipation of the agony you are sure will follow. If you have medication from the doctor, take it immediately; if not, half a teaspoon of table salt plus half a teaspoonful of bicarbonate of soda mixed in a little water often brings some relief. No one knows the reason for this, although bicarbonate of soda is useful in reducing other allergic reactions. A spoonful of honey in a little warm water will not only take away the unpleasant taste of the bicarbonate but will also raise your blood sugar and should help with the nausea and vomiting.

Go to a quiet room, draw the curtains and subdue all light. Try to do the following yoga head-rolling exercise, which will reduce tension in the neck and shoulders, and increase the flow of blood and oxygen to the brain.

1. Sit down with your back straight.
2. Drop your chin forward in toward your neck.
3. Now slowly rotate your head in a clockwise direction, making sure that you are not moving your shoulders or the rest of your body.
4. The slower you do this exercise the better it is. If you feel the desire to yawn or sigh—do so. This is a normal and healthy reaction to this exercise.

5. When you have rotated your head in a clockwise direction six times, change and rotate it in a counterclockwise direction.

6. It is most important that your head be rotated in one direction and then the other.

7. The number of times you do this can be reduced or increased as long as the number is even in each direction.

If you can find a kindly soul to massage your head, scalp, neck, and shoulders, this is the best relief you can obtain. I have found it works better than medication. But do not expect results immediately; a quick five-minute massage is no good at all. This must be a slow and gradual massage: first the shoulders and neck to relax them; then systematically all over the scalp. You must guide the person massaging to the painful points so that he or she can work on them in slow, gentle, circular, outward movements dispersing the pressure and tensions. It may be painful at first, but as the pressure points are relieved and the blood flows more freely, so the pain and nausea will subside.

Always rest after an attack to give the body time to recover.

11

Eating Out

The first thing to remember when eating out, whether it be in a restaurant or at the home of friends, is that you are likely to eat at a different time from your usual mealtime. Even when you have booked a table at a restaurant for 8 P.M. (or your usual dining hour), you will probably find that by the time you have had a drink, looked at the menu, and ordered your meal, it is eight-thirty to eight forty-five or even nine o'clock before you actually *eat* anything. This time factor can be of crucial importance to a migraine sufferer and I suggest that unless you can be absolutely sure you are going to eat early in the evening (for example, when having dinner before going to the cinema or theater), you should always have a high protein snack before going out.

Also remember that if you do eat early in the evening before going on to another engagement, you will need to take another snack in the evening (approximately four hours after the meal) before retiring. If you forget to do this, you could well wake up the next morning with a migraine due to a plummeting of your blood sugar levels after the evening's activities and a fast of perhaps thirteen or fourteen hours.

When accepting invitations to dinner parties, do let your hostess know of your food allergies in advance. For formal occasions when there is a set meal and you cannot find out the menu in advance, take some high protein food, such as a small carton of cottage cheese, with you to eat in the ladies room if you have had to refuse the main part of the meal. Remember, if you are going to dance the night away or do anything energetic, you will need extra snacks.

When eating out, steer clear of small fast food establishments unless you know the menu, because many only supply pork foods such as franks or salami on rye, or ham or cheese sandwiches. It can be embarrassing not to be able to eat anything that is available. Good choices for eating out at lunchtime economically are hamburgers (but only those containing 100 percent ground beef), egg dishes such as omelets or scrambled eggs, and cottage cheese salad. Turkey contains more protein than chicken, so a turkey sandwich would be okay.

If you are eating in a restaurant, you will have to choose your dishes carefully. Anything in a white sauce is suspect, so always ask the waiter to find out if the sauce contains cheese. Many beef dishes or steak in a sauce will have been made with red wine or brandy. Anything cooked with sherry should be avoided, as the heating of wines and sherries seems to increase the amounts of vaso-active amines in them.

Avoid all *gratinéd* dishes, French onion soup, which is usually served with melted cheese as a topping, and minestrone soup, which will probably contain some Parmesan cheese or have it sprinkled on top. When ordering *any* Italian pasta dishes—spaghetti, cannelloni, lasagne—always ask if they contain cheese and ask the waiter not to sprinkle Parmesan cheese on them. Pizzas are not for migraine sufferers and a lot of people will not be able to tolerate salamis, garlic sausages, etc. Most pâtés contain pork meat, fat, or bacon, so must also be avoided. Do not order frankfurters, ham rolls, bacon, and sausages (even beef sausages usually contain some pork!).

Many Chinese dishes contain monosodium glutamate. If this precipitates an attack for you, then it is best to avoid eating in Chinese restaurants.

If you are having a special meal in a restaurant, you may be tempted to have foods that you would not normally include in your everyday diet—so look out for the special foods listed in Chapter 8 that contain unusually high quantities of vaso-active amines. These include raspberries, avocados, pickled herring, eggplant, beans, and shellfish.

Turn down peaches in red wine, pineapple with kirsch, and, of course, chocolate ice cream, profiteroles, éclairs, and cakes.

All liqueurs can be a problem to migraine sufferers, but be especially careful not to have brandy or an orange-based liqueur such as Cointreau or Grand Marnier after your meal.

You can now see how easy it would be to go out for a celebration meal, choosing the following menu, washed down with a bottle of red wine:

Avocado Salad
or
Lima Bean and Bologna Salad
or
Pickled Herring or Pâté

Boeuf Bourguignonne
or
Honey-glazed Virginia Ham
or
Mexican Pork Stew
or
Steak au poivre vert
or
Any variety of Pizza

Raspberries and Cream
or
Chocolate Ice Cream or Cake
or
Chocolate Meringue Torte

Every dish contains migraine precipitant vaso-active amines. You would probably get a very bad attack after a meal like this, but, strangely, you would probably relate the migraine to the excitement and/or stress of going out rather than to the meal itself.

All these warnings about foods you must avoid may leave you wondering what foods you can eat, and how you can produce exciting meals for your family, friends, and yourself without precipitating a migraine. Cheer up! You needn't feel deprived. The recipes and sample menus in the second part of this book will provide a jumbo-sized variety of delicious dishes, from the plain to the exotic, without triggering a migraine attack.

PART II

Recipes—Defense Against Migraine

Recipes

Defense Against Migraine

The following chapter contains sample menus for breakfasts, lunches, dinners, and snacks. By mixing these menus an enormous number of variations for daily eating can be achieved.

Chapters 13 to 15 contain a selection of recipes for breakfasts, main courses, desserts, and snacks. However, a recipe in one category will do just as well in another so that you may find that some of the snack dishes will make delicious breakfasts, or by increasing the portion would make fine main courses. The choice is up to you. These recipes are just to whet your appetite and show that in spite of dietary restrictions you can still eat delicious meals.

First, here are some of the foods that can be a particular problem to migraine sufferers, and ways in which you can modify them or substitute alternatives.

Onions

Many of the recipes contain onions, although there are some migraine sufferers who find that onions can trigger migraine attacks. If you are one of these unlucky people, remember to blanch all onions before using them. This overcomes the problem and you can then proceed with the recipe as directed and suffer no aftereffects.

Blanch by peeling the onions, placing them in cold water, and bringing to the boil. Pour away the water, drain the onions, and use normally.

Chocolate

Under desserts there are a number of "chocolate" recipes. These recipes do not, in fact, contain any chocolate but use the admirable substitute carob powder. Carob tastes very much like chocolate but is much sweeter than unsweetened chocolate powder (cocoa). Dieters take note: it has only a little more than half the calories of chocolate and less than 1 percent fat as against cocoa's 23.7 percent. It is composed largely of carbohydrates but contains natural sugars and a generous supply of B vitamins, calcium, and other minerals. It has a slightly raw taste similar to that of cocoa powder, but this raw flavor disappears if the powder is mixed with a few drops of cooking oil or a little water, then heated for a few minutes to cook it.

If you have a favorite recipe that uses chocolate you may want to adapt it and use carob powder instead. If the recipe originally used cocoa powder, use the same amount of carob powder but reduce the amount of added sugar or sweetener. If the recipe uses sweetened chocolate you will not need to alter the sugar quantity but remember to mix the carob with a little water or oil and cook it for a few minutes, especially when using in icings, fillings, sauces, etc.

Cheese

In many recipes that call for cheese you can substitute cream or cottage cheese, but the result will tend to be somewhat bland, so you may need to increase the seasoning or include additional herbs and spices.

Bananas

Always use bananas that are neither underripe nor overripe.

Citrus Fruits

If you find that citrus fruits precipitate attacks, adapt recipes calling for lemon juice by substituting dry white wine, white wine vinegar, or cider vinegar. Rose's lime juice (which contains little if any real lime juice) is another alternative, as is unsweetened apple juice, or lemon juice made from ascorbic acid, not real lemons. Pineapple is a good substitute for grapefruit, and canned peaches can replace canned mandarins. Garnish drinks with cherries, fresh peach slices, cucumber, or sprigs of mint. Garnish fish dishes with parsley or fennel. Serve duck with black cherries or cranberries instead of oranges.

For fresh juices, try unsweetened pineapple or apple juice or one of the other nonalcoholic beverages mentioned in Chapter 17.

Pork

Veal can be used instead of pork fillet, pork chops, or other pork cuts. For spareribs, use lamb or beef. For pork liver pâté, substitute a calf's liver pâté. In some recipes anchovies can be successfully substituted for ham, salami, or other pork products.

Sugar

White, refined, and artificially colored sugars should be avoided by migraine sufferers; instead use honey, natural brown sugar, maple syrup, or molasses.

Vinegar

White vinegar, preferably white wine vinegar, should be used instead of red wine vinegar or malt vinegar.

12

Sample Menus

Breakfasts

1. Apple juice
   Polynesian Scrambled
     Eggs*
   Whole wheat toast
   Milk or hot beverage
2. Vegetable or V8 juice
   Corned Beef Hash*
   Milk or hot beverage
3. Fresh pears
   Stanley's Breakfast
     Sausage*
   Whole wheat toast and
     butter
   Milk or hot beverage
4. Fresh peaches
   Piperade*
   Whole wheat buttered toast
   Milk or hot beverage
5. Pineapple juice
   Scrapple-style Turkey*
   Whole wheat toast
   Milk or hot beverage

6. Fresh grapes
   Hot Muesli Delight*
   Cottage Cheese Buckwheat
     Squares*
   Milk or hot beverage
7. Fresh apples
   Fish Cakes*
   Milk or hot beverage
8. Grape juice
   Breakfast Hamburgers*
   Milk or hot beverage
9. Fresh pineapple
   Granola Muesli*
   Cottage Cheese Buckwheat
     Squares*
   Milk or hot beverage
10. Fresh strawberries and
      whipped cream
    Egg Nest*
    Milk or hot beverage
11. Watermelon
    Scrambled Tuna and
      Cottage Cheese*

Whole wheat buttered toast
Milk or hot beverage
12. Canned water-packed
    apricots
    Crêpes with Sweet Cheese*
    Milk or hot beverage
13. Cantaloupe
    Pan-fried Porgies*
    Milk or hot beverage
14. Fresh or canned water-
    packed figs
    Golden Apple Pancakes*
    Cottage or Cream cheese
    Milk or hot beverage

Lunches

1. Salad
   Spaghetti Bolognese*
   Fresh grapes
   Beverage
2. Salad
   Shepherd's Pie*
   Fresh apples
   Beverage
3. Salad
   Salmon Soufflé*
   Boiled potatoes and peas
   Beverage
4. Chicken and Mushroom
   Pie*
   Mixed vegetables and
   boiled potatoes
   Fresh pineapple slices
   Beverage
5. Lamb and Apricot
   Kebabs*
   Brown rice

Fresh Peach Ice Cream*
Beverage
6. Salad
   Chicken Brochettes*
   Baked potatoes and carrots
   Beverage
7. Salad Niçoise*
   Whole wheat bread and
   butter
   Apple Cheesecake*
   Beverage
8. Mackerel Provençal*
   Boiled rice
   Aromatic Fruit Salad*
   Beverage
9. Stuffed Bell Peppers*
   New potatoes and carrots
   Honeycomb Mold*
   Beverage
10. Salad
    Broiled Flounder Fillets*
    Potatoes and cabbage
    Carrot Cake*
    Beverage
11. Broiled Calf's Liver*
    Broiled tomatoes and
    french fries
    Fresh peaches
    Beverage
12. Salad
    Chicken and Bean
    Sprouts*
    Brown rice
    Beverage
13. Salad
    Fish Pie*
    Mixed vegetables
    Beverage

14. Salad
    Veal Stew with Parsley
        Dumplings*
    Cherry Almond Tartlets*
    Beverage

Dinners

1. Salad
   Rosemary Lamb
       Casserole*
   Peas and french fries
   Pineapple Cream Custard*
2. Salad
   Barbecued Beef Kebabs*
   Broiled tomatoes
   Baked potatoes in jackets
   Strawberry Shortcake*
3. Salad
   Mexican Chicken in the
       Brick*
   Boiled rice
   Cinnamon Apple Mold*
4. Cream of Watercress
       Soup*
   Brittany Halibut*
   New potatoes and broccoli
   Cherry Tart*
5. Salad
   Swiss Steaks*
   Spinach and french fries
   Pineapple Upside-down
       Cake*
6. Artichoke hearts salad
   Duck with Cranberry-
       applesauce*
   Beetroot and baked
       potatoes in jackets
   Apricot Whip*

7. Salad
   Spiced Ginger Turkey*
   Rice and bean sprouts
   Chestnut Cream with
       Pears*
8. Salad
   Wiener Schnitzel*
   Mushrooms, peas, and
       french fries
   Apricot Kuchen*
9. Cream of Cauliflower
       and Almond Soup*
   Fillets of Sole Margaretta*
   Spinach and french fries
   Strawberry Ice Pudding*
10. Salad
    Roast Chicken with
        Peaches*
    New potatoes and
        broccoli
    Apricot Cheesecake*
11. Salad
    Skillet Lamb with
        Mustard*
    Celery and potatoes
    Chocolate Mousse*
12. Mushroom salad
    Fish Fillets with Egg and
        Applesauce*
    Carrots, zucchini, and
        potatoes
    Black Cherry and Pear
        Tarts*
13. Salad
    Rock Cornish Game Hens
        with Grapes*
    Brussels sprouts and
        sweet potatoes
    Snow Custard*

14. Salad
   Poached Salmon with
      Cucumber Sauce*
   Potatoes and broccoli
   Maple Syrup Chiffon Pie*

Sample Snacks

MIDMORNING

1 Cream Cheese and Walnut
   Sandwich* *or*
1 Scotch Egg* *or*
1 Beef and Mushroom
   Patty* *or*
1 Cream Cheese and Date Filled
   Biscuit* *or*
1 Sweet-sour Chicken
   Drumstick* *or*
1 slice Chicken Loaf* *or*
1 Stanley's Italian Sausage
   Patty*

MIDAFTERNOON

1 Crispy Golden Egg* *or*
1 piece whole wheat bread with
   Sardine Pâté* *or*
1 slice Fish Ribbon Loaf* *or*
1 piece Tuna and Corn Pie* *or*
1 triangle Bumper Decker
   Sandwich* *or*
1 Piquant Cheese Open
   Sandwich*

LATE EVENING

1 Curried Poached Egg* *or*
1 Tuna-stuffed Egg* *or*
1 Chicken Boat* *or*
4–6 Turkey Sesame Balls* *or*
½ portion Cottage Delight* *or*
6 pieces Skewered Cream
   Cheese and Chicken* *or*
1 wedge Spinach Crêpe Stack*

13

Breakfast Dishes

Many people cannot face the thought of eating anything for breakfast. It takes a little time to get used to new eating habits, but remember, breakfast doesn't have to be an elaborate meal, requiring complicated recipes, but should simply be high in protein. Eggs are ideal for a quick, easy and satisfying breakfast. You will probably need to eat 2 eggs to fulfill your protein requirement; these can be hard- or soft-cooked, coddled, poached, or served in a variety of other ways. At low altitudes soft-cooked eggs will take between 3½–4 minutes to cook, depending on whether you put them into cold water and bring to the boil, or directly into boiling water. Hard-cooked eggs take about 12 minutes and coddled eggs 6–8 minutes. At altitudes over 5,000 feet —e.g., Boulder or Denver, Colorado; Butte, Montana; Gallup, New Mexico—increase cooking times to 5–6 minutes for a soft-cooked egg, 15–20 minutes for a hard-cooked egg. The higher, the longer! So you see a nourishing breakfast can be prepared in a very short time.

Golden Apple Pancakes

2 eggs, separated	1 cup yellow cornmeal
1 tablespoon clear honey	1 teaspoon sea salt
2 tablespoons sunflower oil	1 cup grated apples
1 cup milk	Oil for frying

Beat the egg whites until they form peaks. Put the yolks in a separate bowl and stir in the clear honey, oil, and milk. Add the cornmeal, season with salt. Stir until a smooth mixture is obtained. Mix in the grated apples. Gently fold in the beaten egg whites. Cook on a hot oiled griddle or skillet. Serve with maple syrup and whipped cream. Serves 2.

Crêpes with Sweet Cheese

Crêpe batter

1 cup milk	½ teaspoon sea salt
1 cup plus	1 cup all-purpose flour
2 tablespoons water	1 cup whole wheat flour
4 eggs	¼ cup melted butter

Crêpes and filling

Oil for frying	¾–1 cup chopped pecans or
8–10 ounces cream cheese	mixed nutmeats
Honey	

Preheat oven to 375° F. (before frying crêpes).

For the batter: Put all the ingredients for the batter into a food processor or blender in the order given. Process for 1 minute. Scrape any flour left on the sides of the container into the batter and process for 10 seconds more. Leave to stand for 1 hour. The batter should coat a wooden spoon thinly. Add 1 tablespoon more water if needed.

Lightly oil a shallow 6½-inch skillet or crêpe pan. Heat well over moderate heat. Off the heat, pour in enough batter to film the base and swirl around to cover the base completely. Return to the heat for about 1 minute, shaking the pan after 30 seconds to loosen crêpe. Lift edge of crêpe with a spatula; when patchy brown underneath, lift the crêpe on the spatula and turn it over. Cook second side for 30 seconds only. Transfer crêpe to a paper towel.

Repeat until all the batter is used, piling the crêpes on the paper. You should have about 18 crêpes.

Combine the cheese with 4–6 teaspoons honey or to suit your taste. Lay the crêpes flat (do this in batches). Spread 1–1½ tablespoons cheese mixture over each. Roll each crêpe up like a jelly roll. Place the rolled crêpes side by side in a shallow baking pan. Brush well with honey and sprinkle with nuts. Reheat in the oven for 6–8 minutes. Serves 6.

Granola Muesli

1 cup rolled oats	¼ cup chopped almonds
⅓ cup wheat germ	¼ cup chopped dried figs
¼ cup sunflower seeds	¼ cup raisins
¼ cup chopped walnuts	3 apples

Mix the dry ingredients together. Core the apples and slice them with the skin on. Top each portion with apple slices. Serve the muesli with milk and sweeten with maple syrup if desired. Serves 4–5.

Hot Muesli Delight

½ cup cornmeal	¼ cup raisins
3 cups water	1 tablespoon chopped dates
2 apples, finely chopped	1 tablespoon chopped nuts
4 eggs, beaten	

Soak the cornmeal in the water overnight. Next morning add the 2 chopped apples. Bring the mixture to the boil and simmer gently, stirring frequently, until thoroughly cooked (5–10 minutes).

Stir in the beaten eggs. Add the raisins, dates, and nuts, and cook for a few more minutes. Serve hot with honey or maple syrup. Serves 2.

Cottage Cheese Buckwheat Squares

1 cup buckwheat groats	1 teaspoon chopped fresh
1 cup creamed cottage cheese	basil
3 eggs	1 clove garlic, minced
1 tablespoon chopped fresh	Sea salt
parsley	Freshly ground pepper
1 teaspoon chopped fresh	Butter for greasing
chives	

Preheat oven to 400° F.

Cook the buckwheat groats according to the instructions on the package.

Put the cottage cheese in a blender or food processor and blend until smooth. Place in a bowl and add the cooked buckwheat. Mix well.

Separate the eggs. Beat the yolks and combine them with the buckwheat and cheese mixture. Add the parsley, chives, basil, and minced garlic. Mix well and season with salt and lots of freshly ground pepper. Beat the egg whites until stiff and fold into the mixture.

Butter a 10 × 7-inch rectangular pan and pour in the mixture (the depth should be about ½ inch).

Bake for about 30 minutes until the top is lightly browned. Cut into squares to serve. Serves 4.

Piperade

1 small onion	2 tablespoons butter
½ small green bell pepper,	2 eggs
seeded	Sea salt
1 tomato, peeled	Freshly ground pepper

Slice the onion, bell pepper, and peeled tomato very thinly. Melt the butter in a saucepan and gently fry the vegetables for a minute or two. Beat the eggs thoroughly and season with salt and pepper. Add them to the mixture, stirring constantly until the eggs begin to set. They should be the consistency of medium-cooked scrambled eggs. Serve at once. Serves 1.

Scrambled Eggs Petrovitch

4 eggs
Pinch of paprika
Pinch of ground pepper
Sea salt
Chives or scallions (to
  garnish)

1 tablespoon butter
2 slices buttered whole wheat
  toast

Scrambling eggs is quick and easy to do, but you must always cook over a low heat, stir continuously, and serve immediately.

Beat the eggs with a fork or whisk until frothy. Add a pinch of paprika, a pinch of ground pepper, and salt to taste. Chop the chives or scallions and keep on one side.

Put 1 tablespoon butter in a small deep pan (preferably nonstick) and heat until it melts. Add the egg mixture. Cook over very low heat, stirring frequently with a wooden spoon or a fork. In 2–3 minutes the eggs will become "shiny" and semi-solid. Serve at once on hot buttered whole wheat toast and garnish with the chopped chives or scallions. Serves 2.

Pimiento Eggs

½ small red canned pimiento
½ green bell pepper
4 eggs
¼ cup milk
Pinch of cayenne

Pinch of sea salt
Pinch of dry mustard
Dash of chili sauce
3 tablespoons butter
1 small onion, finely chopped

Discard the seeds and chop the pimiento and the bell pepper into small pieces. Beat the eggs, add the milk, and season with the cayenne, salt, and dry mustard. Add a dash of chili sauce.

Put the butter in a skillet and when melted, add the beaten eggs. Stirring all the time, add the chopped onion and mix well. When the eggs are cooked but still soft and creamy, add the pimiento and bell pepper pieces. Stir in for only a minute or two, then serve at once. Serves 2.

Cheesy Scrambled Eggs

2 tablespoons butter
4 eggs
2 ounces cream cheese
A few drops of Worcestershire sauce
¼ teaspoon powdered dried tarragon
Sea salt
Paprika
2 slices buttered whole wheat toast
Chopped fresh parsley (to garnish)

Melt the butter in a saucepan. Beat the eggs and then add the cream cheese, Worcestershire sauce, tarragon, salt, and paprika. Try to soften the cream cheese as much as possible before adding the egg mixture to the melted butter in the saucepan. Proceed as for ordinary scrambled eggs, stirring the mixture all the time. If it thickens too quickly, add a little milk.

When the egg mixture has formed a mass but is still soft and creamy, serve immediately on the toast. Garnish with chopped parsley. Serves 2.

Polynesian Scrambled Eggs

4 eggs
¼ cup fresh coconut milk or unsweetened pineapple juice
4 teaspoons cornstarch or rice flour
4 teaspoons crushed unsweetened fresh or canned pineapple pieces
4 teaspoons grated unsweetened fresh coconut
Dash of salt
Oil for frying
Sesame seeds or toasted grated coconut (to garnish)
Buttered whole wheat toast or corn muffins

Beat the eggs well, then blend in the coconut milk or pineapple juice and the cornstarch. Add the crushed pineapple and grated fresh coconut. Mix well and season lightly with salt.

Pour the mixture into a well-oiled skillet and place over a low to medium heat. Keep stirring with a wooden spoon until a creamy consistency is obtained. Serve hot, sprinkled with sesame seeds or toasted grated coconut, on toast or with corn muffins. Serves 2–3.

Tomato Eggs

1 very small onion
1 tablespoon vegetable oil
1 (8-ounce) can tomatoes
Salt
Freshly ground pepper
Chopped dried or fresh basil
1 tablespoon tomato paste

A few drops of Worcestershire
  sauce
2 hard-cooked eggs plus 2
  hard-cooked yolks
2 slices fried bread or buttered
  whole wheat toast

Chop the onion very finely and fry in the oil over a medium heat until soft but not browned. Drain the canned tomatoes, reserving the juice, and chop them up. Add them to the onions. Season with salt, freshly ground pepper, basil, and tomato paste. Mix together and bring to a boil. Reduce the heat and simmer gently, stirring all the time, adding reserved tomato juice as necessary until you have a thick tomato sauce. Add a few drops of Worcestershire sauce.

Shell the hard-cooked eggs, cut in half, and put the yolks on one side. Cut the whites in thin strips and add them to the tomato sauce. Finely chop the egg yolks.

Cut the fried bread or buttered whole wheat toast into triangles and arrange around the edges of a small plate. Put some of the tomato mixture in the middle, add a layer of the finely chopped egg yolks, then another layer of tomato mixture, and a second layer of chopped yolk. Serve very hot. Serves 2.

Egg Nest

1 medium (4–8 ounce) potato
2 teaspoons butter
2 ounces cream cheese
Sea salt

Freshly ground pepper
½ small onion, finely chopped
1 large egg

Preheat oven to 400° F.

Peel the potato and boil. When cooked, drain and mash with the butter and the cream cheese. Season with salt and pepper and fold in the chopped onion.

Put the mashed potato mixture on a greased flat baking dish arranged like a nest with a hollow in the middle. Break an egg into the hollow and bake on the top shelf of the hot oven for 20 minutes or until the egg white is set. Serves 1.

Plain Omelet

4 eggs
Sea salt

Freshly ground pepper
1 tablespoon butter

Break the eggs into a bowl and beat until frothy; add salt and pepper to taste. Put the butter into a small skillet, using enough to cover the bottom of the pan when melted. Heat until the melted butter begins to smoke. Add the egg mixture quickly and cook over moderate heat, alowing the omelet to set for 1½–3 minutes. As soon as the underside of the omelet is firm, fold the edges into the center using a spatula or wide-bladed knife. Cook for 1–2 minutes more. Divide in half and serve at once. Serves 2.

NOTE: Many different omelets can be easily made by adding sautéed vegetables or other ingredients such as mushrooms, potato, onion, chopped chicken, or flaked fish before folding the omelet.

Corned Beef Hash

½ cup chopped cooked corned
   beef
½ cup mashed potato
1 tablespoon minced onion

¼ cup light cream or stock
Sea salt
White pepper
Butter for greasing

Combine all the ingredients except the butter. Grease a medium-sized heavy skillet with the butter. Put in the hash and cook over low heat, pressing down and stirring from time to time, until browned on the bottom. Fold like an omelet, and turn onto a hot plate. Divide in half to serve. Serves 2.

Kidneys with Mushrooms

8 ounces beef kidney
2 tablespoons all-purpose
    flour
3 tablespoons butter
1 cup chopped mushrooms
1 tablespoon beef bouillon
    granules

Freshly ground pepper
Dried mixed herbs (thyme,
    oregano, sage, marjoram,
    and parsley)
2 slices whole wheat toast
Chopped fresh parsley or
    chives (to garnish)

Cut the kidney into small pieces, discarding all the fat. Roll the pieces in the flour. Heat the butter in a deep pan, add the kidney, and sauté gently, for 3–4 minutes. Add the mushrooms. Dissolve 1 tablespoon beef bouillon granules in a little water. Add it to the pan to make a rich gravy, adding more water if necessary. Add pepper and herbs to taste. Cook for about 10 minutes, then serve on slices of whole wheat toast garnished with chopped parsley or chives. Serves 2.

Stanley's Breakfast Sausage

1 pound chicken (dark meat,
    legs and thighs, removed
    from bone)
1½ teaspoons poultry
    seasoning

1 teaspoon sea salt
¼ teaspoon freshly ground
    pepper
Vegetable oil for frying

Remove the skin and fat from the chicken meat and grind it to a paste in a food processor. Set aside.

Chop the chicken meat in a food processor using the chopper blade, and grind it for about 10 seconds in short bursts. (If you don't have a food processor, cut the chicken meat, with the fat and skin still on, into 1-inch pieces and grind it. If you don't have a grinder, cut the meat with the skin and fat into ¼-inch chunks.)

Mix the fatty paste with the spices and chopped meat. Form the mixture into small patties, moistening it with a little vegetable oil if it is too dry. Heat a little vegetable oil in a skillet and cook the patties slowly, giving them about 5 minutes on each side. Drain on paper towels and serve. Serves 4.

Breakfast Hamburgers

1 pound ground round steak
1 egg, beaten
2–3 tablespoons carrot juice
1 teaspoon French mustard
1 teaspoon sea salt
¼ teaspoon freshly ground pepper

A pinch of ground allspice
Minced fresh parsley (to garnish)
4 hamburger buns, split and toasted

Combine all the ingredients except the minced parsley and buns. Shape into 8 flat patties. Sprinkle a cold skillet with salt. Put in the patties and cook over medium heat, turning once, for about 5 minutes on each side or until done to your liking. Sprinkle with parsley and serve on toasted bun halves. Serves 4.

Scrapple-style Turkey

2 cups cornmeal
2 cups turkey broth
1 small onion, finely chopped
1 large egg, beaten
2 teaspoons sea salt
2½ cups ground cooked turkey meat

1 teaspoon dried sage
½ teaspoon dried thyme
Good pinch of ground cloves
Freshly ground pepper
¼ cup melted butter

In the top of a double boiler, combine the first 3 ingredients. Cook over simmering water until the mush is very thick. Take off the heat. Beat in the egg, then all the other ingredients. Return to the heat, cover, and cook very gently for 40 minutes, stirring occasionally. Turn the mush into a well-greased 9 × 5 × 3-inch loaf pan; press down well and level the top. Chill overnight. To use slice and fry in a little oil. Drain and serve the slices with fried eggs. Makes 8–10 slices.

Creamed Cod Roe

8 ounces cooked cod roe
1 tablespoon butter
1 tablespoon flour
1 cup milk

1 egg yolk, beaten
1 tablespoon grated onion
1 teaspoon white vinegar
3 slices hot toast

Mash the cod roe. Melt the butter in a skillet, blend in flour, then stir in the milk, and cook gently until the sauce thickens. Mix a little hot sauce into the egg yolk, blend, and return to the main sauce. Add the roe, onion, and vinegar. Heat through. Pour over the toast. Serve hot. Serves 3.

Cod Patties

⅔ cup flaked cooked cod
½ cup mashed potato
1 egg, beaten
Sea salt
Freshly ground pepper

Pinch of ground ginger or
paprika
Whole wheat flour
Oil for frying

Combine the flaked fish with the potato and egg; season with the salt, pepper, and ginger. Mix well. Form into 4 round patties and coat with flour. Fry in very hot deep oil until well browned. Drain on a paper towel. Serve hot. Serves 2.

Cod in Scallop Shells

3 tablespoons butter
1¼ cups flaked cooked cod
(skinned and boned)
1 tablespoon whole wheat
flour
1¼ cups milk
1 canned anchovy fillet,
minced

1¼ teaspoons cider vinegar
Dry mustard, cayenne, and
freshly ground pepper
2 large scallop shells
Whole wheat bread crumbs
Chilled, flaked butter

Preheat broiler.

Melt the butter in a saucepan. Add the cod and the flour. Gradually stir in the milk. Season with the minced anchovy fillet and cider vinegar. Sprinkle in a little dry mustard, cayenne, and freshly ground pepper. Cook until the mixture is thick. Grease the scallop shells. Put the mixture into them and top it with a layer of bread crumbs. Dot with flaked butter, and broil until lightly browned. Serves 2.

Sauced Fillets of Haddock

2½ tablespoons melted butter
2 (4-ounce) haddock fillets, skinned
1½ tablespoons all-purpose flour
1 cup hot milk
¼ teaspoon sea salt

⅛ teaspoon paprika
1 teaspoon Worcestershire sauce
1 small gherkin, chopped
1 cup crushed cornflakes
1 tablespoon chilled butter, flaked

Preheat oven to 350° F.

Brush a shallow ovenproof serving dish with a little of the melted butter. Put in the fillets. Put the rest of the melted butter in a pan and stir in the flour. Cook for 2 minutes, stirring, without letting the flour color. Slowly stir in the milk and allow to come to boiling point, still stirring. Add the salt and paprika, Worcestershire sauce, and gherkin. Pour over the fish. Sprinkle the cornflakes on top, and dot with the chilled butter. Bake for 8–12 minutes, depending on the thickness of the fish. Serves 2–3.

Broiled Mackerel with Parsley Butter

1 mackerel, cleaned
Sea salt
Freshly ground pepper
Olive oil
2 teaspoons minced fresh parsley

1 tablespoon butter
2 sprigs parsley (to garnish)

Preheat broiler.

Split the fish along the belly and open it out flat. With a sharp knife or spoon handle, scrape the backbone free of flesh and ease it out. Place the fish, skin side down, in an oiled broiling pan. Sprinkle it with salt, pepper, and olive oil. Broil slowly, without turning, until a creamy curd appears on the flesh, about 12 minutes. Meanwhile, combine the minced parsley and the butter. Place the mackerel on a warmed plate, spread it with the parsley butter, and serve garnished with parsley sprigs. Serves 1.

Pan-fried Porgies

4 whole small (about ¾
  pound each) porgies,
  cleaned
1 cup cornmeal
Sea salt
Freshly ground pepper

½ cup corn oil
1 large clove or 2 smaller
  cloves garlic, finely chopped
¼ cup finely chopped scallions
  (to garnish)

Wash the porgies in cold water, drain and dry. Season the cornmeal with the salt and pepper and roll the porgies in the mixture.

Heat the oil in a large skillet until almost smoking. Add the garlic, then fry the fish until golden brown, about 5 minutes on each side. Use 2 skillets with a small clove of finely chopped garlic in each if there is not room to fry 4 porgies in 1 skillet at one time. Serve hot with a tablespoon of finely chopped scallions scattered over each fish. Serves 4.

Pan-fried Trout

2 (9-inch) trout
1 tablespoon ground almonds
3 tablespoons cornmeal
Sea salt
Freshly ground pepper

1 egg, beaten
Vegetable oil for frying
1 tablespoon chopped fresh
  parsley (to garnish)
Cucumber slices (to garnish)

Wash the trout; drain and dry. Mix the ground almonds and cornmeal and season with salt and pepper. Brush the trout with the beaten egg and then dip them in the cornmeal mixture.

Pour enough oil in a heavy skillet to cover the bottom to a depth of ¼ inch and heat until hot but not smoking. Fry the trout in the oil until browned, about 3–4 minutes each side. Drain on paper towels. Serve sprinkled with chopped parsley and decorated with cucumber slices. Serves 2.

Broiled Trout

4 trout (about ½–¾ pound each)	½ teaspoon French mustard
1 tablespoon sunflower oil	⅔ cup water
2 tablespoons butter	2½ tablespoons cider vinegar
2 tablespoons whole wheat flour	Sea salt
	Freshly ground pepper

Preheat broiler.

Wash and dry the trout; brush with the sunflower oil. Broil the trout near the source of heat for 7–9 minutes until golden brown; about 4 minutes on each side.

Meanwhile melt the butter in a deep pan, take off the heat, and add the flour and mustard, stirring all the time. Gradually add the water and then the vinegar. Season to taste with salt and the freshly ground pepper. Bring to the boil, stirring continuously, and cook for a few minutes. Pour over the trout and serve. Serves 4.

Scrambled Tuna and Cottage Cheese

2 tablespoons butter	½ cup cottage cheese with chives
2 tablespoons all-purpose flour	Sea salt
½ cup milk	Freshly ground pepper
Dash of Worcestershire sauce	Muffins or toast
1 cup flaked canned tuna fish	

Melt the butter, add the flour, and stir over low heat for 2 minutes. Slowly stir in the milk, being careful not to let lumps form, and cook gently until the sauce thickens. Season with Worcestershire sauce. Combine with the flaked tuna and cottage cheese. Mix well. Heat gently without boiling and season. Serve with hot muffins or toast. Serves 3.

Fish Cakes

½ cup mashed potato
2 cups flaked canned tuna fish
2 tablespoons butter
2½ teaspoons chopped fresh
  parsley
Sea salt

Freshly ground pepper
1 small egg
Bread crumbs
Vegetable oil for frying
Parsley sprigs (to garnish)
Tomato slices (to garnish)

Mix the mashed potato with the flaked fish. Melt the butter and combine it with the fish mixture. Add the chopped parsley and season with salt and pepper. Bind the mixture with a little beaten egg and divide into small flat cakes. Coat with the remaining egg, then with bread crumbs. Deep fry in very hot oil, until golden brown. Drain well and serve with sprigs of parsley and slices of tomato. Serves 3–4.

14

Main Courses

Fish

Spanish Cod

4 (4-ounce) pieces cod
¼ cup butter
1 small onion, finely chopped
1 (8-ounce) can tomatoes
2½ tablespoons natural apple
  juice
Pinch of thyme

1 clove garlic, minced
3 teaspoons chopped fresh
  parsley
Sea salt
Freshly ground pepper
Pimiento-stuffed olives (to
  garnish)

Fry the cod pieces in a skillet with a little of the butter for about
15 minutes, turning once. When cooked, place them in an
ovenproof dish and keep hot. Add the rest of the butter to the
skillet, then add the finely chopped onion. Simmer until clear.
Drain the tomatoes, reserving the juice, and cut in small pieces.
Add to the pan with the apple juice, thyme, the garlic, parsley,
and salt and pepper. Add as much of the juice from the tomatoes
as you need to make the sauce smooth and velvety. When the
sauce is cooked, pour it over the fish. Garnish with the pimiento-
stuffed olives. Serves 4.

Indian Curried Haddock

1 clove garlic
6 tablespoons chopped onion
1 tablespoon melted butter or
  vegetable oil
2½ tablespoons curry powder
Sea salt

Freshly ground pepper
4 haddock fillets (about 6
  ounces each)
¼ cup all-purpose flour
2 tomatoes
Cucumber slices (to garnish)

Mince the garlic, then add 2 tablespoons of the chopped onion and the melted butter or vegetable oil and mix with the curry powder to make a paste. Add salt and pepper to taste. Rub this paste over the fish fillets, dust them with flour, then fry in hot fat for 8–10 minutes until cooked, turning them over once.

Wash the tomatoes and chop into small pieces. Mix with the rest of the onion and season with salt and pepper. Serve this mixture cold with the hot fish and garnish with slices of cucumber. Serves 4.

Haddock with Mushrooms

2 pounds fresh haddock fillets,
  skinned
½ cup water
6 tablespoons unsweetened
  apple juice
1 pound mushrooms
2 tablespoons chopped
  blanched onion
2 teaspoons chopped fresh
  parsley

⅓ cup butter
2 tablespoons all-purpose
  flour
1¼ cups hot milk
Sea salt
Freshly ground pepper
1 teaspoon paprika
2 ounces cream cheese
Paprika (to garnish)
Parsley sprigs (to garnish)

Preheat oven to 450° F.

Divide the fish into 4 portions and place in an ovenproof dish. Pour the water and apple juice over it. Slice a few of the mushrooms over the top. Put a lid on the dish and cook in a hot oven for about 15 minutes.

Meanwhile, finely chop the rest of the mushrooms, mix them

with the onion and chopped parsley. Melt ¼ cup of the butter in a saucepan and cook the mushroom mixture gently for 2–3 minutes, then set aside.

When the fish is cooked, drain off the liquid into a saucepan. Keep the fish hot. Boil the liquid for 7 minutes. Melt the remaining butter in a small pan. Add the flour and, stirring all the time, gradually add the hot milk and a good ½ cup of the reduced fish liquid. Simmer for about 6 minutes. Season to taste with salt and pepper, then add the paprika. Add the cream cheese. Stir until smooth.

Stir about ½ of the sauce into the mushroom mixture and pour it into the bottom of a serving dish. Place the fish on top and pour over the remaining sauce. Sprinkle with paprika and garnish with sprigs of parsley. Serve with boiled potatoes. Serves 4.

Brittany Halibut

¼ cup butter	Sea salt
¼ cup chopped onion	Cayenne
¼ cup all-purpose flour	2 pounds halibut, filleted
¼ cup dry white wine	½ cup vegetable oil
2 cloves garlic, minced	1 cup small tomato wedges
2½ tablespoons chopped fresh parsley	Chopped fresh parsley (to garnish)

Preheat oven to 425° F.

Melt the butter in a deep pan and cook the chopped onion in it until it is soft but not brown. Stir in the flour and gradually add the wine, stirring all the time. Simmer for 5 minutes, then add the garlic and the 2½ tablespoons chopped parsley. Season with salt and cayenne. Add a little more wine if the sauce is too thick. Dredge the fish lightly with flour and fry in hot vegetable oil until golden (about 3 minutes on each side). Drain fish on paper towels and then place in a shallow ovenproof dish and cover with the sauce. Make an edging with tomato wedges. Bake in the preheated hot oven for a few minutes until the fish is heated through. Serve sprinkled with chopped fresh parsley. Serves 6.

Broiled Flounder Fillets

½ cup yellow cornmeal
1 teaspoon wheat germ
1 teaspoon fennel seeds
Sea salt
Freshly ground pepper
4 flounder fillets (4–5 ounces each)

Parsley sprigs (to garnish)
Cucumber slices (to garnish)
Young green onions (to garnish)

Preheat broiler.

Combine the cornmeal, wheat germ, and fennel seeds in a bowl and season with the salt and pepper. Dip each fillet in the mixture, so that both sides are coated. Arrange the fillets in the broiler pan and slowly brown them in the broiler, giving them about 10 minutes on each side.

Garnish with parsley sprigs, cucumber slices, and bunches of young green onions. Serves 4.

Mackerel Provençal

2 medium onions
4 mackerel (about 1 pound each), filleted and unskinned
2 cups chopped drained canned tomatoes
1 large clove garlic, minced
½ teaspoon ground fennel seeds

½ teaspoon dried basil
½ teaspoon dried oregano
1½ tablespoons olive oil
12–16 pitted green olives
½ teaspoon sea salt
Freshly ground pepper

Preheat oven to 350° F.

Thinly slice the onions. Place the mackerel fillets and sliced onions in alternate layers in a casserole.

Combine the rest of the ingredients in a small bowl, and season with the salt and pepper. Mix well. Pour this sauce over the fillets in the casserole.

Bake uncovered for about 1 hour, or until the fish is tender. Serves 6–8.

Broiled Salmon Steaks

2 (¾-inch-thick) salmon
 steaks
2 teaspoons grated onion
1 tablespoon white vinegar
3 tablespoons melted butter
½ teaspoon sea salt

Pinch of freshly ground
 pepper
¼ teaspoon dried marjoram
½ tablespoon chopped chives
1 tablespoon chopped fresh
 parsley

Preheat broiler.

Place the salmon steaks on a foil-lined broiler pan. Combine the remaining ingredients. Pour half the mixture over the salmon. Broil about 2 inches from the source of heat for about 4 minutes. Turn the salmon over. Pour the remaining seasoning mixture over them. Broil 6 minutes longer. Serve hot, with the juices poured over. Serves 2.

Salmon Salad

1 (15-ounce) can salmon
½ small sweet red bell pepper,
 seeded and chopped

2½ tablespoons sweet chutney
⅓ cup pimiento-stuffed olives
Bunch of watercress or lettuce

For the dressing

⅔ cup light cream
2½ tablespoons white wine
 vinegar
1 tablespoon chopped fresh
 chives

Salt
Freshly ground pepper

Drain off any liquid from the salmon and flake the flesh into a bowl. Add the bell pepper, chutney, and pimiento-stuffed olives. Mix together well. Line a serving plate with the watercress or lettuce and pile the salmon mixture in the center.

For the dressing: Make a dressing for the salmon by blending together the light cream, vinegar, and chives. Season with salt and freshly ground pepper. The dressing can either be spooned over the salmon or served separately in a dish. Serves 4.

NOTE: Tuna or swordfish may be substituted for salmon.

Poached Salmon with Cucumber Sauce

¼ cup butter
1 small onion, finely chopped
1 medium carrot, chopped
5 cups water
1¼ cups dry white wine
1 teaspoon sea salt

6 white peppercorns
4 small salmon pieces (about
    4 ounces each)
Chopped green onion (to
    garnish)

For the sauce

1¼ teaspoons minced onion
2½ tablespoons white wine
    vinegar
¾ teaspoon salt

A few drops of Tabasco
⅔ cup whipped cream
1 cucumber

Melt the butter in a deep pan. Add the vegetables and cook slowly for 5 minutes without browning. Add the water, wine, salt, and peppercorns. Simmer for another 5 minutes. Put the salmon pieces into the pan and simmer very slowly for about 20 minutes, then lift out carefully and drain. Allow to get quite cold and then remove the skin.

For the sauce: Mix the onion with the vinegar, salt, and Tabasco. Fold lightly into the whipped cream. Peel and grate the cucumber. Drain thoroughly and then fold into the sauce. Chill.

To serve: Pour or spoon the sauce over the salmon pieces and garnish with chopped green onion. Serves 4.

Salmon Soufflé

1 pound potatoes
1 (8-ounce) can red salmon,
    drained
2 eggs
2 tablespoons butter

1¼ tablespoons chopped fresh
    parsley
Sea salt
Freshly ground pepper

Preheat oven to 375° F.

Peel and boil the potatoes. Mash the salmon. Separate the eggs, add the yolks to the salmon, reserving the whites. Mash the butter and potatoes, then add the salmon mixture and parsley. Season

with salt and pepper. Beat the egg whites until stiff, then fold into
the salmon mixture. Place in a greased 1-quart soufflé dish and
bake for 30–35 minutes. Serve with a green salad. Serves 4.

Salmon Florentine

2 tablespoons butter
2 tablespoons all-purpose
   flour
¾ cup milk
¼ teaspoon dry mustard
Pinch of sea salt
1–2 drops of Tabasco

1 cup chopped cooked
   spinach (squeezed dry)
1 tablespoon grated onion
2 tablespoons diced cucumber
1 cup drained and flaked
   cooked or canned salmon

Preheat oven to 400° F.

Melt the butter, add the flour, and stir for 2 minutes over low
heat. Slowly stir in the milk and cook gently until the sauce
thickens. Season with the dry mustard, a little salt, and Tabasco.

Combine the spinach with the grated onion and cucumber.
Place in 2 well-greased individual casseroles. Put half the salmon
on top of the mixture in each casserole, and spoon the sauce
over. Bake for about 15 minutes until well heated through.

This dish can be prepared for baking the night before; keep
covered in the refrigerator. Serves 2.

Crunchy Fillets of Sole

2 fillets of sole (about 5–6
   ounces each)
Dash of sea salt
2 tablespoons sweet chutney

½ cup fresh whole wheat
   bread crumbs
1 tablespoon sesame seeds
2 tablespoons melted butter

Preheat oven to 350° F.

Skin fillets if necessary. Lay side by side in a buttered roasting
pan. Sprinkle with salt, then spread with chutney. Mix together
the crumbs and sesame seeds and sprinkle over the fillets; press
lightly. Sprinkle with melted butter. Bake for 10–12 minutes until
fish is tender. Serve at once. Serves 2.

Fillets of Sole Margaretta

⅔ cup sunflower oil

4 large fillets of sole, about 8 ounces each

Sea salt

Freshly ground pepper

½ cup mushrooms, finely chopped

1 shallot or small onion, finely chopped

2 tablespoons butter

¼ cup canned whole corn, drained

Paprika

Chopped fresh parsley (to garnish)

Put the oil in a skillet and heat. Season the fillets with salt and pepper, fry gently in the oil until cooked (about 3 minutes each side). Drain well, place on a serving dish and keep warm. Add the mushrooms to the shallot or onion. Gently cook this mixture in the butter until tender, but do not brown. Stir in the canned corn and season with salt and pepper.

Pour the sauce over the fish, sprinkle with paprika, and decorate with chopped fresh parsley. Serves 4.

Fish Pie

2 tablespoons butter

3 shallots or small onions, finely chopped

⅔ cup dry white wine

1½ pounds mixed white fish, skinned and boned

6 ounces puff pastry

For the sauce

2 tablespoons butter

¼ cup flour

Fish liquid

⅔ cup light cream

Sea salt

Freshly ground pepper

Preheat oven to 400° F.

Heat 2 tablespoons butter in a pan and fry the chopped shallots. Add the wine. Break the fish into pieces and add to the mixture. Cook for about 5 minutes. Lift fish out of the liquid and put into a 1½-quart deep baking dish or casserole. Keep the liquid aside.

For the sauce: Melt 2 tablespoons butter, remove from heat, and stir in the flour. Gradually add the reserved fish liquid and cream. Season with salt and freshly ground pepper. Cook slowly until thickened, stirring constantly. Pour over the fish.

Cover the pie with the puff pastry and bake for 20 minutes, then reduce the heat to 375° F. and bake for another 10–15 minutes. Serves 4.

Fried Whiting

2 whiting (about ¾ pound each)
¼ teaspoon dried thyme
¼ teaspoon crushed dried rosemary
¼ teaspoon sea salt

Freshly ground pepper
½ cup milk
¼ cup cornmeal
2 teaspoons wheat germ
¼ cup butter

Clean the fish, rinse and dry. Remove the heads and fins. Sprinkle the herbs inside, and season well. Dip the fish in the milk, then roll in cornmeal and wheat germ. Heat the butter in a large skillet and fry the fish, turning once, until tender and browned on both sides. Serves 2.

Fish Fillets with Egg and Applesauce

1 pound white fish fillets, skinned
Sea salt
Freshly ground pepper
2 tablespoons butter
2 tablespoons all-purpose flour

1 cup milk
¼ small apple, peeled and grated
2 hard-cooked eggs, chopped
1 tablespoon apple juice
1 teaspoon mild white vinegar

Sprinkle the fillets with salt and pepper, and wrap in cheesecloth. Lay them on a trivet in a kettle over simmering water. Cover, and steam for 8–12 minutes, depending on the thickness of the fish. (Fish still frozen will take a bit longer.)

Meanwhile, melt the butter in a pan, stir in the flour, and cook gently, stirring, for 2 minutes. Slowly, add the milk, and stir until the sauce thickens. Season lightly. Stir in the grated apple, chopped egg, apple juice, and vinegar. Heat through and then spoon over the fish. Serve at once. Serves 3–4.

Baked Fish Fillets

Small white fish fillets (about 1–1¼ pounds)	Sea salt
	White pepper
2–4 tablespoons butter	Chopped chives (to garnish)

Preheat oven to 400° F.

Wash fresh fillets or thaw frozen fillets, and skin. If necessary, cut into slices about ¾ inch thick. Place the fish fillets in a shallow ovenproof dish that just fits them, greased with a little of the butter. Season with salt and pepper and dot with the rest of the butter. Cover the dish with a lid or aluminum foil. Bake in oven for 15–20 minutes. Garnish with chopped chives. Serves 3–4.

Poultry & Game

Chicken Breasts Italian Style

1 tablespoon vegetable oil	16 pimiento-stuffed olives
4 chicken breasts	2½ tablespoons cornstarch
1 pound potatoes, peeled	¼ cup dry white vermouth
2 cups raw whole button mushrooms	2½ tablespoons tomato paste
	1 teaspoon dried oregano
1 cup chopped onion	2 cups chicken stock

Preheat oven to 350° F.

Heat the vegetable oil in a large skillet and lightly fry the chicken breasts until brown on both sides. Drain, reserving the remaining oil in the skillet. Place the breasts in an ovenproof casserole dish. Cut the potatoes into small sticks. Wash but do not peel the mushrooms. Place the potatoes, mushrooms, and chopped onion in the skillet and fry until golden brown. Add them to the chicken in the casserole. Sprinkle the pimiento-stuffed olives over the top.

Blend the cornstarch with the vermouth and combine with the tomato paste and oregano. Blend the mixture into the stock and mix well. Pour over the chicken. Put a lid on the casserole and cook in the moderate oven, until tender, for 45 minutes–1 hour. Serves 4.

Chicken Vermouth

4 chicken breasts	Sea salt
2 tablespoons butter	Freshly ground pepper
2½ tablespoons sunflower oil	8 ounces button mushrooms
⅓ cup dry vermouth	2½ tablespoons cornstarch
1¼ cups chicken stock	Watercress or parsley sprigs
1¼ tablespoons chopped fresh	(to garnish)
tarragon	

Preheat oven to 350° F.

Skin the chicken breasts if desired. Melt the butter in a large skillet and add the sunflower oil. Fry the chicken pieces in the mixture for about 15 minutes until they are nicely browned on both sides. Pour in the vermouth and set alight. Shake the pan gently until the flames die down. Slowly stir in the stock, tarragon, and seasoning and bring to the boil. Transfer to a large casserole dish with a lid and bake in the medium oven for about 40 minutes.

Wash and dry the mushrooms and add them to the casserole, making sure they are covered by the liquid. Bake for another 10 minutes. Test the chicken to see if it is cooked. If clear liquid runs from the meat when it is spiked with a skewer, it is done. Remove the chicken pieces and put on a large serving dish. Cover with aluminum foil and keep warm. Pour the juices from the casserole into a saucepan and thicken them with cornstarch blended into a thin paste with a little of the juices. Boil for a few minutes, stirring constantly. Spoon the sauce over the chicken and serve. Garnish with watercress or parsley sprigs. Serves 4.

Chicken Breasts with Dates and Carrots

¼ cup chopped onion
1 clove garlic, minced
½ cup sunflower oil
1½ cups chopped dates
1 cup finely shredded carrots
2 cups cooked rice
½ teaspoon crushed dried
  rosemary

½ cup chopped almonds
2 teaspoons honey
Sea salt
Freshly ground pepper
6 chicken breasts, boned

Preheat oven to 350° F.

Sauté the onion and garlic in the oil until clear but not brown. Combine the dates, carrots, cooked rice, rosemary, almonds, and honey with the onion mixture. Season with salt and freshly ground pepper. Mix with a wooden spoon.

Spoon equal amounts of the mixture onto each chicken breast. Turn over the edges and skewer. Place in a well-oiled shallow baking dish or pan. Brush the top of each one with oil. Bake for about 1½ hours. Serves 6.

Chicken with Cashew Nuts

1 (3½-pound) whole cooked
  chicken
2 tablespoons butter
½ cup raw cashews
1 medium onion, chopped
1 apple, peeled and diced
8 ounces potatoes, peeled and
  diced

2½ teaspoons mild curry
  powder
1¼ cups chicken stock
⅓ cup golden raisins
Sea salt
White pepper
1¼ cups milk
2½ tablespoons heavy cream

Remove the cooked meat from the chicken. Cut into bite-sized pieces. Melt the butter in a large skillet and fry the nuts until golden brown. Add the chopped onion, diced apple, and potatoes. Fry gently for about 5 minutes. Add curry powder, the chicken pieces, stock, and golden raisins. Cook gently for 30 minutes. Add salt and pepper to taste. Add milk slowly, stirring all the time. Add the cream just before serving. Serves 4.

Chicken Brochettes

4 boneless chicken breasts
(about 4 ounces each)
2½ tablespoons apple juice
1 large onion, peeled
⅔ cup softened butter
⅓ cup finely chopped fresh
parsley

Sea salt
Freshly ground pepper
12 apricot halves (if dried,
soak overnight)
Pitted ripe black olives
1¼ tablespoons olive oil

Preheat broiler.

Skin the chicken breasts and cut them into 1½-inch pieces. Place on a plate and pour the apple juice over them. Cut the onion into chunky pieces. Cream the butter, and add the parsley, salt, and freshly ground pepper. Drain the apricot halves and fill the hollows with the parsley butter. Drain the olives.

Thread the pieces of chicken breast, onion, apricots, and olives alternately on skewers. Brush the whole lot with a little olive oil. Grill in the broiler pan 3–4 inches from the heating element without a rack for about 20 minutes, turning and basting frequently. Serve with the juices spooned over. Serves 4.

Chicken Cassata

1¼ cups chicken stock
1¼ tablespoons gelatin
½ teaspoon Tabasco
3 tablespoons cider vinegar
6 tablespoons mayonnaise
12 ounces cooked chicken
meat, diced

2½ teaspoons very finely
chopped chives
3 stalks celery, chopped
1 small green bell pepper,
seeded and diced
1 red apple, diced
Salad greens

Put the chicken stock into a deep pan, sprinkle the gelatin into it, and dissolve over low heat. Do not boil. Add the Tabasco and cider vinegar. Leave to cool but *not* set. Beat the mayonnaise into the mixture gradually and when it begins to thicken, fold in the chicken, chives, celery, pepper, and apple. Turn into a mold that has been rinsed but not dried. Chill until set. Unmold and serve on a bed of salad greens. Serves 4.

Deviled Chicken

1 (3½–4-pound) roasting
  chicken
1 cup flour
1 teaspoon barbecue spice
1 teaspoon sea salt
1 teaspoon paprika
1 teaspoon chili powder
1 tablespoon prepared
  mustard

2 teaspoons chili sauce
2 tablespoons cider vinegar
½ teaspoon Tabasco
1 egg, beaten
⅓ cup evaporated milk
½ cup butter

Preheat oven to 350° F.

Divide the chicken into 8 serving pieces. Combine the flour, barbecue spice, salt, paprika, and chili powder in a large bowl. Mix thoroughly.

In a second bowl combine the mustard, chili sauce, cider vinegar, Tabasco, egg, and evaporated milk. Mix well.

Dip each chicken piece first into the seasoned flour, then into the mustard mixture, and then again into the seasoned flour.

Melt the butter in a roasting pan and arrange the chicken pieces in it, skin side down. Bake in the medium oven for 25 minutes, then turn the pieces over, baste, and bake for another 25 minutes. Serves 4.

Roast Chicken with Peaches

1 (3½-pound) chicken,
  including giblets
Sea salt
Freshly ground pepper
3 cups fresh whole wheat
  bread crumbs
1 small onion, finely chopped

1 slice Canadian bacon, finely
  chopped (optional)
1 (15-ounce) can sliced
  peaches in syrup
2 teaspoons honey
2½ tablespoons vegetable oil

Preheat oven to 425° F.

Remove the liver and giblets and wash and dry the chicken. Put the liver and giblets in a pan. Season with salt and pepper and cover with water. Boil gently for 20 minutes.

Put the bread crumbs in a bowl and mix in the finely chopped onion. Add bacon, if desired. Remove the cooked chicken liver from the pan, discarding the water. Mash the liver and add it to the mixture in the bowl. Season with salt and freshly ground pepper.

Drain the peaches, reserving the liquid; add them to the mixture together with a tablespoon of the syrup from the can and a teaspoon of honey. Make the mixture damp enough for it to stick together, adding more peach syrup if necessary. Stuff the chicken with this mixture and put it in a roasting pan. Rub a teaspoon of honey over the skin, sprinkling liberally with salt and pepper. Pour the remainder of the peach syrup over, then add the vegetable oil. Roast the chicken in the hot oven for 30 minutes. Turn the oven down to 375° F. and continue to cook for another hour until nicely browned and completely cooked. Baste frequently. Serves 4.

NOTE: For a change, add a piece of ginger, finely chopped, from a jar of candied ginger in syrup, to the peach stuffing mixture and pour a little of the ginger syrup over the chicken before roasting.

Chicken and Bean Sprouts

2 cups chicken stock	2 cups finely chopped skinned
1 tablespoon butter	cooked chicken
⅓ cup whole wheat flour	1 teaspoon curry powder
½ cup chopped carrots	1 teaspoon soy sauce
½ cup chopped onion	1 tablespoon raisins
½ cup chopped celery	1 cup bean sprouts
½ cup chopped sour apple	2 cups hot cooked brown rice

Put the stock and butter in a large pan and bring to the boiling point. Measure 1¼ cups of the stock into a jug. Stir the flour into the stock in the pan without letting lumps form. Gradually stir in the stock in the jug. Continue stirring until the sauce thickens, then add the vegetables and apple. Simmer for 20 minutes or until the vegetables are soft. Stir in the chicken, curry powder, soy sauce, and raisins, and simmer 5 minutes longer. Add the bean sprouts and stir around well, then serve over hot brown rice. Serves 4.

Chicken and Apricots

6 fleshy chicken pieces
1 medium onion, chopped
Sea salt
Freshly ground pepper
½ teaspoon ground ginger
1 teaspoon ground cinnamon
1 tablespoon dried mixed
  herbs

2½ tablespoons chicken fat
8 ounces dried apricots,
  soaked overnight
1 pound tart apples
2–3 tablespoons honey
1 tablespoon apple juice

Put the chicken pieces, onion, a little seasoning, and the spices and herbs in a large saucepan. Add the fat and just enough water to cover the ingredients. Bring slowly to the boil. Lower the heat to simmering point, and simmer gently, half covered, until the chicken is tender, about 1 hour. Add the drained apricots after the first 15 minutes. By the end, the cooking liquid should be reduced a good deal, to a rich sauce.

Meanwhile, peel, core, and slice the apples. When the chicken is tender, remove the pieces and keep warm. Add the apples, honey, and apple juice to the sauce, stir in gently and simmer for 15 minutes or until the apples are just tender. Adjust the seasoning. Return the chicken and reheat in the sauce without boiling. Serves 6.

Broiled Chicken

4 chicken breasts
¼ cup apple juice
Melted butter for brushing
Sea salt
Freshly ground pepper

8 canned peach halves in
syrup or 4 slices canned
pineapple in syrup plus a
few spoonfuls of syrup from
the can

Preheat broiler.

Sprinkle the chicken breasts with the apple juice, then brush them with melted butter and season with salt and pepper. Place chicken portions in broiler pan, skin side down. Broil about 6 inches from the source of heat for 10–12 minutes. Turn the pieces over and broil for a further 10–15 minutes, skin side up.

Baste with melted butter from time to time. For the last 5 minutes cooking, place 2 peach halves or 1 slice of pineapple on each chicken breast, and spoon a little of the fruit syrup over the top of them. Serves 4.

Chicken with Almonds

4 chicken breasts	¾ teaspoon clear honey
Vegetable oil	3 drops of Worcestershire
⅔ cup chicken stock	sauce
2½ teaspoons cornstarch	2 tablespoons slivered
¾ teaspoon dry mustard	almonds, toasted
¼ cup apple juice	

Preheat oven to 375° F.

Arrange chicken breasts in a single layer in a shallow baking dish. Brush with oil. Pour the chicken stock over them and bake in the moderate oven for about 40 minutes. Remove chicken from juice and keep warm.

On the top of the stove blend the cornstarch and mustard with the apple juice, honey, and Worcestershire sauce and stir into the bubbling juices in the baking dish. Keep stirring until a smooth sauce is obtained.

Place the chicken pieces on a serving dish, pour the sauce over them, and sprinkle the toasted almonds on top. Serves 4.

Mexican Chicken in the Brick

1 (3½-pound) chicken	2 tablespoons curry powder
1 clove garlic	2 tablespoons unsalted
1 small apple, peeled	peanuts or cashew nuts
1 small onion	2 tablespoons raisins
1–1½ cups cooked rice	2 tablespoons vegetable oil
2 tablespoons clear honey	Sea salt
1 teaspoon ground ginger	Freshly ground pepper

Remove giblets from chicken, and rinse inside and out. Pat dry.

Finely chop the garlic, apple, and onion. Add them to the cooked rice with 1 tablespoon honey, the ginger, and 1 tablespoon of the curry powder. If you prefer hot curries, add extra curry powder. Mix in the nuts and raisins. Combine with 1 tablespoon oil. Stuff this mixture into the chicken until quite full; you may not use all of it. Place the chicken in a chicken brick. Dribble a little oil over it and 2 teaspoons honey. Sprinkle well with 2 teaspoons of curry powder and a little salt and pepper. Put any stuffing left over around the chicken in the bottom of the brick; sprinkle with 1 teaspoon curry powder and remaining oil and honey.

Place the chicken brick into a *cold* oven and set the oven to 470° F. (fiercely hot). Cook for 1½–2 hours, until the meat comes away from the bone easily. Serve with rice and a tossed green salad. Serves 4.

Sweet and Sour Chicken

2½ tablespoons sunflower oil	½ teaspoon chili powder
4 chicken breasts	2½ tablespoons cornstarch
1¼ cups chicken stock	1¼ tablespoons soy sauce
1 (8-ounce) can pineapple pieces	⅔ cup white wine vinegar
½ cup sliced and seeded green bell pepper	1 tablespoon blackstrap molasses
½ cup sliced and seeded sweet red bell pepper	Sea salt (optional)
	Freshly ground pepper

Preheat oven to 350° F.

Put the oil in a large skillet and fry the chicken on both sides until browned. Drain the chicken on paper towels and put in a 1½-quart casserole dish. Pour the chicken stock over. Put a lid on the casserole and cook in the moderate oven for about 45 minutes.

Pour the juices off into a saucepan. Keep the chicken pieces warm. Add the pineapple and peppers to the juices in the saucepan and simmer for 5 minutes. Blend the chili powder with the cornstarch, then blend with the soy sauce, vinegar, and molasses. Add to the stock, stirring all the time until the sauce thickens and clears. Add salt and pepper to taste.

Pour the sauce over the chicken breasts and serve on a bed of freshly boiled long-grained rice. Serves 4.

Polynesian Chicken

2½ tablespoons vegetable oil	1 tablespoon cornstarch
4 chicken breasts	¼ cup water
1 (15-ounce) can pineapple chunks in natural juice	2 tomatoes or 1 sweet red bell pepper
1 tablespoon soy sauce	1 green bell pepper
2–3 stalks celery, chopped	

Put the oil in a large skillet and brown the chicken portions on both sides. Drain chicken on paper towels and keep warm. Drain pineapple and reserve the juice. If necessary, add water to the juice to make ⅔ cup. Add the juice and soy sauce to the skillet. Stir in the chopped celery and simmer, covered, for 20 minutes. Blend the cornstarch with the ¼ cup water and stir into the mixture in the skillet. Bring to the boil. Add pineapple chunks. Cut tomatoes into 8 wedges or, if using sweet red bell pepper, discard seeds, cut into rings, and add to the mixture. Cut green bell pepper into rings, discarding seeds, and add to the skillet. Place the chicken pieces on top and simmer for another 10–15 minutes until the chicken is tender. Serve with rice. Serves 4.

Chicken and Mushroom Pie

1 (3-pound) cooked chicken	2 cups milk
1 medium onion	1 tablespoon chicken bouillon granules
1 clove garlic	
3 tablespoons butter	⅓ cup flour
1 cup mushrooms cut into quarters	8 ounces plain pastry

Preheat oven to 425° F.

Cut the chicken into chunky pieces. Finely chop the onion and garlic. Put the butter into a deep skillet and gently fry the onions, garlic, and mushrooms in it for 2–3 minutes. Meanwhile, warm the milk in a saucepan (do not boil) and dissolve the bouillon granules in it.

Stir the flour into the butter which is frying the onions and mushrooms. Gradually add the milk mixture, stirring all the time, until it is smooth and thick. Add the chicken.

Turn into a 9-inch deep baking dish. Allow to cool, then cover with the pastry and bake in the hot oven for 20–25 minutes. Serves 4.

Spiced Chicken Drumsticks

2–3 chicken drumsticks per person

2 tablespoons curry powder (per 6 drumsticks)

Vegetable oil

Clear honey

Sea salt

Preheat boiler.

Wipe the chicken drumsticks and dry them. Mix the curry powder with a little vegetable oil, then roll each leg in the mixture until it is completely covered. Arrange the chicken drumsticks in a broiler pan and dribble clear honey over them. Sprinkle with salt. Place 6 inches from heat source and broil for 10–15 minutes turning once until they are crisp on the outside. They will turn very dark brown. Take care the honey does not make them burn. Serve with rice or bread and a mixed salad.

Turkey Breast Fillets in Cream

1 pound turkey breast fillets

2½ tablespoons sunflower oil

½ cup finely chopped onions

2 teaspoons paprika

2 cups chicken or turkey stock

1 green bell pepper, seeded and sliced in strips

½ cup small pasta shells

Sea salt

Freshly ground pepper

⅔ cup heavy cream

1 teaspoon cornstarch, blended with 1 teaspoon water

Chopped fresh parsley (to garnish)

Cut the turkey fillets into small strips. Heat the oil in a pan and gently fry the onion until golden. Add the turkey and paprika to the pan. Raise the heat, stir and fry quickly to seal the turkey pieces. Do not burn the onion. Stir in the stock and bring to the boil. Add the pieces of green bell pepper and pasta and season with salt and pepper.

Put a lid on the pan and simmer gently for 15–20 minutes until the turkey and pasta are tender. Stir in the cream and thicken with the blended cornstarch. Serve garnished with chopped parsley. Serves 4.

Spiced Ginger Turkey

4 turkey drumsticks (about 9–10 ounces each)

3 ounces preserved ginger plus 2½ tablespoons syrup from jar

1 (15-ounce) can pineapple pieces, drained

¾ cup soy sauce

4½ tablespoons white wine vinegar

¾ cup dry white wine

A few drops of angostura bitters

Sea salt

Freshly ground pepper

Finely chopped scallions and chives (to garnish)

Cut the skin off the turkey drumsticks and make cuts in the flesh so that the turkey absorbs the marinade.

Place the turkey pieces in a shallow ovenproof dish in 1 layer. Slice the ginger into small pieces and mix with the drained pineapple pieces. Add the soy sauce, wine vinegar, white wine, a few drops of angostura bitters, and ginger syrup, and mix well. Season with salt and pepper and spoon the whole mixture over the turkey. Cover and marinate overnight.

Next day, preheat oven to 425° F., and cook in a covered dish in the hot oven for about 1 hour until the flesh is tender. Baste as necessary. Serve garnished with finely chopped scallions and chives. Serves 4.

NOTE: Chicken can be cooked the same way, but you will need to allow more chicken drumsticks per person than with turkey.

Rock Cornish Game Hens with Grapes

2 Rock Cornish game hens	⅔ cup white grapes
2½ tablespoons sunflower oil	1 tablespoon cornstarch
¾ cup chicken stock	1 egg yolk
3 ounces dry white wine	2½ tablespoons heavy cream
Sea salt	Chopped fresh parsley (to
Freshly ground pepper	garnish)

Cut the birds in half and remove the backbones and the outside skin. Put the oil in a skillet and lightly fry the bird halves in it until they are golden brown on both sides. Now pour the stock and wine over the birds and season with the salt and freshly ground pepper. Bring the mixture to the boil and simmer gently for about 25 minutes until the meat is tender.

Meanwhile, wash the grapes, cut them in half, and remove the seeds. Blend together the cornstarch, egg yolk, and cream. When the birds are cooked, take them out of the skillet, drain them, and keep them warm on a serving dish.

Add the cornstarch mixture and the grapes to the juices in the skillet. Cook gently without boiling until the sauce thickens, 5–10 minutes. Stir frequently. Add seasoning if necessary. Pour the sauce over the birds, garnish with the parsley, and serve immediately. Serves 2.

NOTE: The same recipe can be used for squabs.

Duck with Cranberry-applesauce

2 sweet apples	3 cups raw cranberries
About ¼ cup apple juice	1 (4–5-pound) duck
2 teaspoons honey	

For stuffing

½ cup sage and onion stuffing mix	¼ cup apple jelly
	¼ cup cranberry-applesauce
1 duck liver	Sea salt
1 small onion	Freshly ground pepper

Preheat oven to 425° F.

Peel and slice the apples and put in a saucepan. Add 2 teaspoons apple juice, the honey, and just enough water to cover the fruit. Simmer gently until fruit is just tender. Add the cranberries. Simmer 5 minutes or until they pop. Put aside.

Make the stuffing mix according to the instructions on the packet. Meanwhile cook the duck liver in a little water for 15–20 minutes. Mince the onion, and add it to the stuffing mix. When the liver is cooked, discard liquid, chop the liver and add it to the stuffing mixture together with 2 tablespoons of the apple jelly and ¼ cup cranberry-applesauce. Season lightly.

Stuff the duck with the above mixture. If there is too much, bake the extra stuffing separately in a small ovenproof dish. Sprinkle the duck with salt and pepper. Spoon the remaining 2 tablespoons of apple jelly over it. Put it in a baking pan with 3 tablespoons of apple juice. Do *not* use any fat or oil.

Put into the hot oven for 30 minutes, then reduce the heat to 375° F. and cook for 1½ hours until the duck is brown and crisp on the outside, and sweet and succulent within. Serve with the reheated cranberry-applesauce handed separately. Serves 4.

Duck with Black Cherries

1 (4–5-pound) duck, including giblets
Sea salt
Freshly ground pepper
1 small onion
2 cloves garlic
1 (15-ounce) can pitted black cherries

⅓ cup whole wheat bread crumbs
4 teaspoons clear honey
1¼ tablespoons minced fresh sage
1 cup apple juice
2 tablespoons cornstarch
Watercress sprigs (to garnish)

Preheat oven to 425° F.

Take out the giblets and wash and dry the duck. Cook the giblets in a little water with salt and pepper for 10–15 minutes.

Meanwhile, mince the onion and 1 clove garlic. When the giblets are cooked, reserve the liquid, take out the liver and mash it up with the onions and the minced garlic. Drain the cherries, reserving the liquid. Chop ⅓ of the cherries and add them to the liver mixture. Bind the stuffing together with bread crumbs, a little of the water the giblets were cooked in, and 2 teaspoons of clear honey. Season with salt and pepper and mix in the sage.

Now stuff the duck with the liver mixture and put it in a roasting pan. Combine half the reserved cherry juice with about ⅔ cup of apple juice and a little water. Pour over the duck. Rub a teaspoonful of honey over the duck's skin and sprinkle liberally with salt. Prick the skin in several places with a fork. Put into the hot oven for 30 minutes, then reduce heat to 375° F. and cook for another 1½ hours until the duck is brown and crisp on the outside and sweet and juicy inside, with all the fat drained out of it.

Mix the cornstarch with a little of the remaining cherry juice, then put it in a saucepan with the rest of the cherries. Heat gently and add the rest of the cherry juice and the last teaspoon of honey. Crush the remaining garlic and add the juice to the pan. Season with salt and pepper. Stirring all the time, add remaining apple juice. Add water if necessary to keep the sauce from getting too thick.

Serve the roast duck garnished with watercress sprigs. Serve the sauce separately. Serves 4.

Baked Rabbit in Cream

1 rabbit (about 3–4 pounds)	¾ cup light cream
⅓ cup French mustard	Sea salt
¼ cup vegetable oil	Freshly ground pepper

Preheat oven to 350° F.

Skin and divide rabbit into portions and place in a roasting pan. Cover the rabbit pieces thickly with the mustard. Dribble the oil over the top. Cover with aluminum foil and bake for 1–1½ hours, until well browned.

When cooked, put the rabbit pieces on a dish and keep hot. Stir the cream into the pan juices over a low heat. Season with salt and pepper. Cook for 2–3 minutes, stirring constantly. Serve the rabbit with the sauce poured over. Serves 4.

Meat

Swiss Steaks

1 (1-pound) piece round
   steak, 1½ inches thick
Sea salt
Freshly ground pepper
2 tablespoons flour
1 tablespoon butter for
   greasing

1 (14-ounce) can Italian
   tomatoes
1 medium onion, sliced
1 medium carrot, sliced
1 small potato, peeled and
   diced

Preheat oven to 300° F.

Cut the meat into serving portions. Season the pieces with salt
and pepper, and pound the flour into it with a meat mallet. Heat
a heavy skillet, and grease it with butter. Put in the meat, and
brown it well on both sides. Transfer the meat to a 1½-quart casserole and cover with the tomatoes. Add the other vegetables.
Season well. Cover and bake at 300° F. for 1¾ hours or until the
meat is very tender. Remove the meat to a warmed serving dish.
Skim any fat off the sauce in the casserole, and spoon the vegetables and a little sauce over the meat. Serves 3.

Stuffed Bell Peppers

2 tablespoons vegetable oil
1 small onion, minced
1 clove garlic, minced
¾ cup ground beef
¾ teaspoon Worcestershire
   sauce
¾ teaspoon oregano
Sea salt

Freshly ground pepper
1 (8-ounce) can Italian plum
   tomatoes, with juice
4 mushrooms, sliced
2 tablespoons tomato paste
2 green or red sweet bell
   peppers (about 6 ounces
   each)

Preheat oven to 425° F.

Put the oil in a saucepan together with the minced onion and garlic; cook until soft and yellow but do *not* brown. Add the ground beef, Worcestershire sauce, oregano, salt, and pepper. Drain the tomatoes, and reserve the juice. Add the tomatoes to the mixture in the pan together with the mushrooms and tomato paste. Add a little of the reserved tomato juice if necessary to prevent the mixture from sticking, but try to keep it as dry as possible. Simmer gently for about 30 minutes, stirring frequently.

Cut the tops off the bell peppers and remove the seeds. Place the bell peppers in a dish small enough to keep them in an upright position. Stuff the bell peppers with the above mixture and replace the tops.

Add a little water to the bottom of the dish to prevent the bell peppers from sticking. Put in a hot oven and cook for 25–35 minutes. Serves 2.

Barbecued Beef Kebabs

For the sauce

2 tablespoons vegetable oil
2 small cloves garlic, finely chopped
2 tablespoons ground ginger
1 tablespoon ground cumin
1 tablespoon honey
1 tablespoon white cornmeal

2½ tablespoons white wine vinegar
1 tablespoon tomato paste
1¼ teaspoons soy sauce
1½ teaspoons unsweetened dried grated coconut

For the kebabs

9 ounces beef fillet
Sea salt
Freshly ground pepper

Worcestershire sauce
A few drops of vegetable oil

For the sauce: Heat 2 tablespoons vegetable oil in a pan with the chopped garlic. Do not brown. Add the ground ginger, cumin, and honey. Mix thoroughly and add the cornmeal. Stirring all the time, add the vinegar, tomato paste, soy sauce, and coconut. Simmer gently for 1 hour, adding enough water to keep the sauce of pouring consistency. Do not allow to burn.

For the kebabs: Preheat broiler and cut the beef fillet into cubes and place on 2 skewers. Sprinkle with salt, freshly ground pepper, and a few drops of Worcestershire sauce. Dribble over a few drops of vegetable oil. Place in the broiler about 4 inches from the source of heat, for 10–15 minutes, turning once or twice so that the meat is cooked on both sides.

Pour the sauce over the cooked kebabs and serve on a bed of rice or with pieces of fresh bread and a green salad. Serves 2.

Shepherd's Pie

2½ tablespoons vegetable oil	¼ teaspoon marjoram
2 medium onions, finely chopped	Sea salt
	Freshly ground pepper
1 pound ground round steak or chuck	1 tablespoon beef bouillon granules
2 cups chopped mushrooms	2–3 drops brown food coloring
1 (14-ounce) can tomatoes, with juice	1½ pounds potatoes
¼ teaspoon dried thyme	3 tablespoons butter
¼ teaspoon dried sage	

Put the oil in a pan and gently fry the onions without browning them. When they are transparent, add the ground steak and mushrooms. Mash the canned tomatoes with the juice and gradually add them to the steak mixture in the pan. Stir with a wooden spoon. Add the herbs, salt, freshly ground pepper, and the bouillon granules. Cook for 30–45 minutes until the mixture is moist but not runny. Add a few drops of coloring.

Preheat broiler.

Meanwhile peel the potatoes and boil them in water to cover. When cooked, drain off the water, add the butter, season with salt and pepper, and mash until smooth and creamy.

Put the ground steak mixture into a 9-inch-diameter deep baking dish or casserole; it should almost fill the dish. Cover with the mashed potato and put the pie into the broiler, about 4 inches from the heat source, for 7–10 minutes until well browned. Serves 4.

Spaghetti Bolognese

2½ tablespoons olive oil
1 large onion, finely chopped
1 large clove garlic, minced
1 pound ground round steak
1 (14-ounce) can peeled
    tomatoes
1 tablespoon finely chopped
    capers
½ cup pitted ripe olives

1 teaspoon dried basil
3 tablespoons tomato paste or
    purée
1 teaspoon honey
Sea salt
Freshly ground pepper
1 pound spaghetti
½ cup cottage cheese

Heat the oil in a saucepan and gently fry the chopped onion and garlic until yellow and translucent. Add the ground beef. Drain the tomatoes and reserve the juice. Add the tomatoes to the pan, chopping them into pieces with a fork.

Add the finely chopped capers, olives, basil, tomato paste or purée, and honey. Stir well, add salt and freshly ground pepper and enough of the reserved tomato juice to maintain a fairly thick consistency. Cook for 35 minutes.

Meanwhile, cook the spaghetti in a large pot of lightly salted boiling water to which you have added a couple of drops of oil. Do not overcook. It should be just tender but *not* sticky. This faint "bite" is what the Italians call *al dente*.

Serve on separate plates with the spaghetti making a nest for the sauce. Top each serving with a tablespoon of cottage cheese. Serves 4.

Wiener Schnitzel

6 (5-ounce) veal cutlets
⅓ cup dry white wine
2 eggs
A few drops of sunflower oil
¾ cup whole wheat flour

Sea salt
Freshly ground pepper
1½ cups whole wheat bread
    crumbs
½ cup butter

Trim cutlets and flatten with a heavy mallet. Pour the white wine over the meat and leave for about an hour, turning several times.

Break the eggs in a dish and mix with a few drops of oil and a few drops of water. Mix the flour with the salt and pepper. Dip the marinated veal in the flour first, then into the egg mixture. Lastly, coat well with bread crumbs.

Heat the butter in a large skillet and fry the crumbed slices slowly until golden brown, turning once. They should sizzle when you put them in the skillet. Serve with boiled potatoes or french fries and with individual salads. Serves 6.

Veal Stew with Parsley Dumplings

Flour

12 ounces boneless veal stew
   meat, cut in 1-inch cubes

Fat for frying

2 cups tomato juice

1 teaspoon sea salt

2–3 drops of Tabasco

Pinch of white pepper

½ cup diced peeled potatoes

¼ cup sliced celery

¼ cup chopped onion

For dumplings

½ cup flour

1 teaspoon baking powder

1 tablespoon minced fresh
   parsley

1 teaspoon minced chives

¼ teaspoon sea salt

¼ cup milk

1 tablespoon melted butter

Flour the meat. Brown it in a little fat in a large saucepan. Add the tomato juice and seasonings. Cover and simmer very gently for 1 hour. Add the vegetables and cook 20 minutes longer. Meanwhile, make the dumplings.

For the dumplings: Combine the dry ingredients, and moisten with the milk and butter.

Drop spoonfuls of the mix on the stew, cover, and simmer for 15 minutes. Serve from the pot. Serves 3.

Broiled Calf's Liver

¼ cup butter

1 beef bouillon cube,
   crumbled

8 ounces calf's liver, sliced

Chopped fresh parsley (to
   garnish)

Preheat broiler.

Cream the butter until soft and add the crumbled bouillon cube. Wash and trim the liver and lay the slices side by side in a broiler pan. Spread half the butter mixture over the liver slices and broil about 4 inches from heat source for about 5 minutes. Turn slices over, spread remaining savory butter over them, and broil about 5 minutes more. Serve with the juices spooned over and garnish with chopped parsley. Serves 2.

Skillet Lamb with Mustard

1 pound lean lamb from fillet
  end of leg
About 4–5 tablespoons Dijon
  mustard
¼ cup butter

A few drops of sunflower oil
½–1 cup beef or lamb broth
8 sprigs watercress (to
  garnish)

Cut the meat into 4 equal-sized pieces. Discard all fat. Spread the mustard thickly on both sides of each piece. Melt the butter in a skillet and add a few drops of oil. Fry the fillets slowly, turning once, until browned on the outside and pale pink in the center— approximately 15–20 minutes. Take the pieces out of the skillet and keep warm. Add a little broth to the juices in the skillet and simmer gently for 5 minutes. Pour over the lamb pieces, and serve garnished, with watercress sprigs. Serves 4.

NOTE: Although a lot of mustard is used in this recipe, the completed result does not taste hot.

Lamb and Apricot Kebabs

2½ tablespoons sunflower oil
1¼ tablespoons dry white wine
1 (15½-ounce) can apricot
  halves, in unsweetened juice
¼ cup finely chopped onion
1 clove garlic, minced

½ teaspoon dried thyme
Bay leaves
1 pound lean lamb from fillet
  end of leg
Sea salt
Freshly ground pepper

Make a marinade of the oil, wine, 2½ tablespoons of the apricot juice, onion, garlic, and herbs. Cut the meat into bite-sized cubes and put them in the marinade for 2–3 hours. Drain the apricot halves discarding the juice, and dip them in the marinade for 2 minutes. Season with salt and freshly ground pepper.

Preheat broiler.

Drain meat and fruit and skewer alternately meat, fruit, bay leaf, meat, fruit, bay leaf, etc. Place in broiler pan 4 inches from heat source and broil for about 15 minutes, turning once. Serve on a bed of boiled long-grained rice. Serves 4.

Rosemary Lamb Casserole

⅓ cup butter
A few drops of vegetable oil
4 pounds boned lamb, cut into small pieces
½ cup flour
2–3 onions, sliced
2 cups sliced celery
3 cups sliced cored peeled apples

2½ cups lamb or veal stock
1¼ cups apple juice
Sea salt
Freshly ground pepper
Crushed dried rosemary
2 cups thinly sliced peeled potatoes
Watercress (to garnish)

Preheat oven to 350° F.

Put ¼ cup of the butter and a little vegetable oil in a skillet and heat. Roll the lamb pieces in the flour and brown them quickly in the heated fat. Drain and put meat into a deep casserole.

Put the onions and celery, together with the sliced apples, in the skillet. Fry lightly. Then put the onion, celery, and apples in the casserole on top of the meat. Pour the stock and apple juice over the dish and season well with salt and pepper and crushed dried rosemary.

Top with a layer of thinly sliced potatoes and dot with remaining butter.

Bake in the moderate oven for about 1½ hours. Serve garnished with watercress.

Roast Lamb with Rosemary

½ shoulder of lamb (about
   2–2½ pounds)
2½ tablespoons vegetable oil
Crushed dried rosemary

Sea salt
Freshly ground pepper
1 clove garlic
1¼ cups dry white wine

Preheat oven to 425° F.

Wipe and dry the lamb and place in a roasting pan. Pour the vegetable oil over the meat, then sprinkle it heavily with dried rosemary, salt, and pepper. Chop the garlic very finely and add it to the wine, then pour into the roasting pan. Roast the meat for 30 minutes in the center of the preheated oven, then turn down to 375° F. to cook for another 1½ hours. If it is beginning to cook too quickly and burn turn oven down to 350° F. When ready, it should be brown with crisp fat and succulent meat. Serves 4.

15

Desserts

Apple Cheesecake

½ cup finely crushed graham
 crackers
⅔ cup dry muesli mix
¼ cup butter
2 tablespoons brown sugar
1 (8-ounce) package cream
 cheese
1½ teaspoons ground
 cinnamon
⅔ cup heavy cream

2 eggs, separated
2½ teaspoons clear honey
1 tablespoon gelatin
5 tablespoons water
6 tablespoons clear honey
1 red eating apple (to garnish)
⅓ cup halved seedless grapes
 (to garnish)
Walnut halves (to garnish)

Grease an 8-inch round layer pan. Combine the crushed graham crackers and dry muesli. Melt the butter in a saucepan and add the cracker mixture and the brown sugar. Stir well. Press the mixture firmly over the base of the pan, and place in the refrigerator for 10–15 minutes.

Meanwhile, beat the cream cheese, cinnamon, and heavy cream together, gradually adding the egg yolks and 2½ teaspoons of honey. Beat until a smooth texture is obtained.

Dissolve the gelatin in 3 tablespoons of warm water. When it is cool but not set, stir it into the cheese mixture. Beat the egg whites, gradually adding 3 tablespoons of the clear honey. Beat until egg whites stand in peaks, then gently fold into the cheese mixture. Pour the cheese mixture into the prepared pan and chill until set.

Decorate the top of the cake with unpeeled freshly sliced apples, seedless grapes, and walnut halves. Quickly make a glaze with the remaining clear honey dissolved in 2 tablespoons of water and brush over the fruit and nuts. Serves 6.

Cinnamon Apple Mold

2 pounds eating apples	3 tablespoons gelatin
1¼ cups water	⅓ cup cold water
1¼ cups apple juice	2 eggs
½ cup clear honey	2 teaspoons ground cinnamon
2 cloves	

Peel and core apples, and cook with the 1¼ cups water, apple juice, honey, and cloves until soft.

Soak the gelatin in the ⅓ cup of cold water for a few minutes, then heat until dissolved. Beat the eggs and put aside.

Discard the cloves. Purée the apples. Strain the gelatin and stir into the apple purée. And 1 teaspoon of the cinnamon and fold in the beaten eggs.

Pour into serving dish and leave to set. Before serving, sprinkle the top with the remaining cinnamon. Serve with whipped cream. Serves 6.

Almond Fingers

4 ounces plain pastry dough	⅓ cup honey
Butter for greasing	2½ teaspoons ground rice
2 tablespoons apricot	(Cream of Rice)
preserves	⅓ cup chopped skinned
1 egg white	blanched almonds
¾ cup ground almonds	2 drops of almond extract

Preheat oven to 350° F.

Roll out the pastry into a 7-inch square and leave for 30 minutes. Grease a 7-inch square baking pan and line the bottom with the pastry. Spread the apricot preserves over the pastry. Beat the egg white stiffly. Combine the remaining ingredients and mix well. Fold in the beaten egg white. Spread this mixture evenly over the preserves. Bake for about 25 minutes until lightly browned. Remove pan from oven. When nearly cool, cut into fingers and finish cooling on a wire rack. Serves 4.

Almond and Apricot Open Pie

½ cup butter
2 cups all-purpose flour, sifted
⅓ cup brown sugar, lightly
  packed
½ cup ground almonds

3 egg yolks, beaten
About 2 tablespoons cold
  water
1¼ pounds fresh apricots

Preheat oven to 375° F.

Rub the butter into the sifted flour and add sugar and ground almonds. Bind the dough with the beaten egg yolks and about 2 tablespoons cold water. Roll out dough to ⅛ inch thick and line a 9-inch pie plate with it. Keep remaining dough aside.

Halve and pit the apricots and arrange them in the pastry shell. Use the remaining dough to make pastry strips and arrange in a lattice over the apricots.

Bake for about 30 minutes. Serves 6.

NOTE: Use the leftover egg whites for the Apricot Kuchen.*

Apricot Kuchen

8 ounces rich piecrust dough
3 egg whites
1 cup ground almonds

1 pound fresh apricots
¾ cup warm melted honey
½ cup heavy cream

Preheat oven to 400° F.

Grease a 10-inch round shallow baking pan and line with the dough. Beat the egg whites until stiff and fold in the ground almonds. Spread this mixture over the dough.

Cut apricots in half and remove the pits. Arrange apricots, cut side up, on top of almond mixture. Bake in the hot oven for 10 minutes, then reduce heat to 350° F. and cook for 45 minutes longer until the pastry is cooked. Brush with a little of the still warm melted honey.

Whip the cream. Serve the kuchen warm and pass the whipped cream and the remaining warm honey syrup separately. Serves 4–6.

Apricot Mousse

1 cup firmly packed dried
    apricots
2½ teaspoons gelatin
¼ cup apple juice

2 teaspoons clear honey
¾ cup heavy cream
1 egg white
Slivered almonds (to garnish)

Soak the apricots in cold water until swollen. Put apricots in a pan, cover them with the liquid they have been soaking in, and simmer with a lid on the pan until tender, about 20 minutes.

Soak the gelatin in a small bowl with the apple juice. Drain the apricots, saving ½ cup of the liquid. Put the fruit in a food processor or blender with the ½ cup apricot liquid, gelatin mixture, and honey and blend until smooth.

In separate bowls, whip the cream and beat the egg white until stiff. Fold the cream into the blended mixture, then fold in the beaten egg white. Refrigerate to set and decorate with slivered almonds. Serves 4.

Apricot Whip

¾ cup apricot purée
    (preferably made from
    fresh apricots)
¼ cup honey
3 egg whites

¾ cup heavy cream
2–3 teaspoons vodka
1 teaspoon almond extract
½ cup water

Put the apricot purée in a pan and heat. Add the honey and stir until blended in, keeping the purée simmering all the time.

Beat the egg whites until stiff. Fold into the hot purée in spoonfuls, whipping with a fork. Beat until the mixture is thick. Leave to cool.

Whip the cream with the vodka and almond extract until it stands in peaks, then fold it into the almost-cold apricot mixture with the water. Spoon into serving dishes and chill. Serves 4.

Apricot Sherbet

1 cup dried apricots	¼ cup apple juice
6 tablespoons honey	1 egg white

Place the apricots in water to soak overnight, then poach them in the soaking liquid for about 20 minutes in a covered pan.

Strain off the liquid and make up to 1¼ cups with water, return to the apricots in the pan, and add the honey. Bring to the boil and boil for 2–3 minutes. Allow to cool. Then purée the apricots with a little of the cooled syrup and the apple juice if possible in a food processor or blender. Stir the rest of the liquid into the purée and freeze the mixture until mushy. Beat the egg white until stiff.

Put the mushy mixture into a chilled bowl and beat well until smooth. Fold in the stiffly beaten egg white and return to the freezer. Freeze until firm. Transfer to the refrigerator for about 1 hour before serving. Serves 6.

Apricot Cheesecake

3 cups dried apricots	5 teaspoons gelatin
1 cup water	⅓ cup dry white wine
6 tablespoons clear honey	1 cup cottage cheese
1 cup crushed graham crackers	1 (8-ounce) package cream cheese
¾ cup butter, melted	1 (14-ounce) can evaporated milk
¼ teaspoon ground cinnamon	8 canned apricot halves (to garnish)
¼ teaspoon ground cloves	
¼ teaspoon ground allspice	
¼ teaspoon ground coriander	

Soak the dried apricots overnight in cold water. Drain and simmer them in 1 cup water with ¼ cup honey for about 20 minutes until cooked. Chop the apricots coarsely and keep aside.

Put the crushed crackers into a bowl and mix with the melted butter, spices, and 2 tablespoons honey.

Use ¾ of the crumbs to line the base of an 8½-inch loose-bottomed cake pan. Refrigerate to set.

Dissolve the gelatin in the wine and put it in a food processor or blender with both cheeses and the evaporated milk. Blend until smooth. Fold in the coarsely chopped apricots. Pour mixture over the crumb base, scatter the remaining cracker crumbs on top, and refrigerate to set. Turn out upside down to serve. Decorate the cheesecake with well-drained canned apricot halves arranged cut side down. Serves 6.

Snow Custard

6 eggs, separated	1½ teaspoons vanilla extract
1¼ cups milk	½ cup crushed slivered
1¼ cups light cream	almonds
½ cup clear honey	Chopped fruits (to garnish)

Beat the egg yolks well. Mix the milk, cream, ¼ cup honey, and ½ teaspoon vanilla extract in the top of a double boiler. Beat in the egg yolks. Make a custard with these ingredients by stirring them gently over simmering water until thickened and smooth. Pour into a large flat shallow serving dish. Cover with waxed paper and set aside to cool.

Warm 2 tablespoons of the honey. Beat the egg whites until frothy. Add the warmed honey and crushed slivered almonds gradually while beating and continue beating until the mixture is stiff and glossy. Pour about 1½ inches water into a 10-inch skillet and flavor it with the remaining vanilla extract and honey. Bring slowly to simmering, stirring to dissolve the honey. Then put in large heaped spoonfuls of the meringue (the size of a small apple). Poach a few at a time until firm underneath, turn over carefully with 2 spoons, and poach the second side. Place the meringues on the custard, either around the edge or piled in the center. Decorate with chopped fruits. Serves 4–6.

Cherry Almond Tartlets

1 cup all-purpose flour
½ cup ground almonds
¼ cup clear honey
6 tablespoons butter
1 cup fresh red cherries

⅔ cup water
2½ teaspoons cornstarch
2½ tablespoons kirsch
¼ cup chopped blanched
    almonds

Preheat oven to 400° F.

Make an almond pastry dough with the flour, ground almonds, 2 tablespoons of the honey, and the butter. Use ⅔ of the dough to line two 4-inch pie plates. Make thin strips out of the remaining dough and keep aside.

Pit the cherries and cook with the remaining honey and water until tender. Drain well, reserving the juice.

Blend the cornstarch with the kirsch, and stir into the reserved juice. Bring the mixture to the boil, stirring constantly. Add the cherries and almonds. Allow to cool, then spoon into the pastry shells. Use the reserved strips to make a lattice covering for each tartlet. Bake for 20–25 minutes. Cool in the pans. Serves 2.

Cherry Tart

6 ounces plain pastry
3 tablespoons clear honey
2 tablespoons all-purpose
    flour

½ teaspoon ground cinnamon
1 (15-ounce) can pitted black
    cherries
2 tablespoons butter

Preheat oven to 425° F.

Roll out ⅔ of the pastry dough and use it to line a greased 7-inch pie plate. Put the honey, flour, cinnamon, and ⅔ cup cherry juice from the can into a saucepan and cook gently until the mixture thickens and boils.

Meanwhile drain the cherries. Pour the mixture from the pan over the cherries and allow to cool a little before piling the cherry mixture into the pastry shell. Dot with butter. Dampen the edges of the pastry. Roll out the rest of the pastry and use to cover the pie. Seal the edges and make 2–3 slits in the top crust. Bake until browned in the hot oven, 35–45 minutes. Serves 4–6.

Chestnut Cream with Pears

1 pound French or Italian
 chestnuts
About 1 pint milk
Honey

¼ cup raisins
2 large fresh sweet pears
2 ounces cream cheese
½ cup heavy cream

Gash the flat side of each nut. Cover with boiling water and bring back to boiling point slowly. Boil for 10–15 minutes. Drain, discarding liquid. Shell and remove inner brown skins while still hot. Drop the nuts as soon as they are peeled into enough scalding hot milk to cover them all. Simmer for 20–30 minutes until the nuts are tender. Purée in a blender or food processor the drained chestnuts, with enough honey to sweeten to your taste, only just until smooth. Add a little of the cooking milk if the mixture is very stiff. Do not overprocess. Fold in the raisins.

 Peel the pears, halve them lengthwise, and cut out the cores with a teaspoon. Cut a sliver off the rounded side of each half to make it rest level. Arrange the pears in a serving dish cut side up and pile 1 tablespoon of cream cheese in the core hollow of each pear half. Cover with the chestnut purée. Whip the cream and swirl on top. Serves 4.

Black Cherry and Pear Tarts

2¼ cups all-purpose flour
⅞ cup clear honey
6 tablespoons butter
1 egg, lightly beaten
A few drops of vanilla extract
⅔ cup water
2 sweet pears (about 8 ounces
 each) or 1 (15-ounce) can
 pears, drained

8 ounces dark dessert cherries,
 pitted
4 ounces cream cheese
1 tablespoon milk
2 teaspoons arrowroot

Preheat oven to 400° F.

Sift the flour into a bowl and add 2 teaspoons of the honey and the butter. Mix together and then add the lightly beaten egg and vanilla extract. Knead well until it becomes a pliant dough, then put in a cool place for 30 minutes.

Take eight 2½ × 1¼-inch muffin pan cups and grease them. Roll out the dough and cut out rounds to fit the pans. Line each cup with dough, then with greased aluminum foil. Bake the shells empty for 8–10 minutes. Remove aluminum foil and allow to cool. Remove from the cups.

Meanwhile put the water and ½ cup honey into a pan, and heat until it becomes syrupy. Peel, halve, and core the pears if fresh and gently poach them in the syrup for 15 minutes or until they are tender. Remove from the heat and add the cherries. Cover the pan and allow to cool.

Put the cream cheese, the milk, and remaining honey into a bowl and beat until creamy. Spoon a little cheese mixture into each tart shell. Drain the fruit, reserving the syrup. Cut up the pears, and spoon fruit over cheese mixture.

Slowly, blend the reserved syrup with the arrowroot in a small pan, until smooth. Bring to a boil, stirring gently. Take off the heat when the sauce has thickened and cleared. Use it to glaze the fruit in the tarts. Makes 8 tarts.

Golden Carrot Cookies

¾ cup butter	1 cup mashed cooked carrots
1 cup clear honey	2 cups all-purpose flour, sifted
1 egg, beaten	½ teaspoon sea salt
½ teaspoon vanilla extract	2 teaspoons baking powder

Preheat oven to 350° F.

Cream the butter and honey until light and fluffy. Add the egg, vanilla, and mashed carrots. Beat well. Sift the flour, salt, and baking powder together. Add to the carrot mixture a little at a time, blending well after each addition. Drop the mixture by teaspoonfuls 2 inches apart on ungreased cookie sheets. Bake for 20 minutes. Makes 72 small cookies.

Carrot Cake

4 medium carrots	1¼ cups all-purpose flour
⅔ cup pecan halves	½ teaspoon sea salt
2 eggs	1 teaspoon baking soda
½ cup clear honey	1 tablespoon ground
⅓ cup salad oil	cinnamon
⅔ cup milk	

Preheat oven to 300° F.

Grease a 9-inch square cake pan. Grate the carrots and nuts. Beat the eggs, honey, oil, and milk together until blended. Add the carrots and nuts. Sift together the flour, salt, soda, and cinnamon. Combine quickly with the carrot mixture. Do not overbeat. Turn the mixture into the prepared pan, and level the top. Bake for 1 hour. Cool in the pan for 15 minutes, then turn out on a wire rack. Serve warm with chilled cream or cool and cover with frosting. Serves 8.

Date Cream

1¾ cups milk	¼ teaspoon salt
½ cup thinly sliced dates	1 egg, beaten
⅓ cup cornstarch	2 tablespoons honey
¼ cup chilled light cream or	½ teaspoon vanilla extract
half-and-half	

Scald the milk in the top of a double boiler. Add the dates, and simmer for 1 minute. Blend the cornstarch with the light cream and salt and stir into the milk. Cook until the mixture thickens, stirring constantly. Reduce the heat to a very slow simmer, cover and cook for 10 minutes. Meanwhile beat the egg and honey together. Add to the hot mixture and stir for 1 minute. Remove from the heat.

Fold in the vanilla extract. Pour into a serving dish. Cool, covered with waxed paper and aluminum foil. Then chill for 1–2 hours. Serve with swirls of whipped cream on top. Serves 4–6.

Fresh Peach Ice Cream

4 fresh peaches	¼ cup apple juice
1 (14-ounce) can sweetened	¾ cup heavy cream
condensed milk	Slivered almonds (to garnish)

Peel and slice 3 of the peaches, discarding the pits, and put them in a food processor or blender with the condensed milk, apple juice, and cream. Blend until the mixture is quite smooth and very creamy. Pour into ice trays or a shallow plastic container and fast-freeze until firm.

Take out of freezer and put in refrigerator for 30 minutes before serving. Decorate with slices of remaining fresh peach and slivered almonds, and serve. Serves 6.

Pineapple Upside-down Cake

3 tablespoons warmed clear	½ cup milk
honey, plus extra for glazing	⅓ cup butter
12 slices fresh pineapple	½ cup dark brown sugar,
6 ounces crumbled pound	lightly packed
cake	3 eggs, separated
¾ cup ground almonds	

Preheat oven to 350° F.

Line a 10-inch square cake pan with greased baking paper. Spread the honey over the bottom and arrange 9 pineapple slices on top. Chop the remaining slices.

Combine the chopped pineapple, cake crumbs, and ground almonds in a bowl, and pour the milk over them. Cream the butter and sugar, beat in the egg yolks, then combine with the cake crumb mixture. Beat the egg whites until stiff, then fold them into the batter. Turn the batter into the prepared pan.

Bake for 45–55 minutes in the moderate oven. Turn out upside down. Glaze with a little extra warmed honey, and serve warm. Serves 6–8.

Coconut Mold

3 eggs, separated
2 cups milk
1 cup grated fresh coconut
1 envelope gelatin

3 tablespoons honey
¼ teaspoon sea salt
1½ teaspoons vanilla extract

Combine the egg yolks, 1 cup of the milk, the grated coconut, gelatin, honey, and salt in a saucepan. Cook gently until the gelatin is dissolved, stirring constantly. Take off the heat and leave to stand for about 20 minutes. Add the remaining milk and chill until the mixture begins to thicken. Beat the egg whites with the vanilla extract until they reach stiff peaks. Fold the coconut mixture into the egg whites. Spoon into a 6-cup mold and chill until firm. Unmold and serve. Serves 6.

Pineapple Delight

1 small (6-fluid ounce) can
    evaporated milk
6–8 macaroons
1 (15-ounce) can crushed
    pineapple, drained

1 cup cold thick custard
Toasted slivered almonds (to
    garnish)

Boil the evaporated milk in the unopened can covered with water for 20 minutes. Cool. Meanwhile crush the macaroons and put in a serving bowl. Cover the macaroons with a layer of the crushed pineapple, reserving the rest. Whip the evaporated milk and add it to the cold custard, whip again thoroughly, then fold in the rest of the crushed pineapple.

Pile this mixture onto the macaroons and serve decorated with toasted slivered almonds. Serves 4.

Pineapple Cream Custard

2 (15-ounce) cans pineapple
    pieces
1 thick slice (about 1 ounce)
    pound cake, broken in
    pieces

1 whole egg
1 egg yolk
¾ cup heavy cream
3 tablespoons milk
2 tablespoons brown sugar

Preheat oven to 325° F.

Drain and crush the pineapple pieces and put a little in each of 4 individual custard cups. Then divide the pound cake among the 4 cups. Beat the whole egg with the extra yolk. Add the cream and milk, and beat until smooth.

Pour the mixture into the dishes. Put the dishes in a baking pan half filled with water. Bake in a moderate oven for 30–35 minutes until set. Chill well and serve sprinkled with the brown sugar. Serves 4.

Curried Fruit Medley

8 fresh apricots
4 sweet pears
1 cup cubed fresh pineapple
¼ cup butter

Curry powder (about 2
  teaspoons)
¼ cup clear honey

Preheat oven to 325° F.

Skin, halve, and pit the apricots. Peel, halve, and core the pears, then cut into chunks. Combine the apricots and pear chunks with the pineapple cubes. Grease an 8-inch bake-and-serve shallow pan. Arrange the fruit in it.

Melt the butter. Mix in the curry powder and honey. Heat until the honey is fully melted. Pour the mixture over the fruit. Bake for about 40 minutes. Serve hot with chilled whipped cream. Serves 6.

Butterscotch Creams

2 tablespoons butter
⅓ cup brown sugar, lightly
  packed
1¼ cups milk

1¼ tablespoons cornstarch
About 1 tablespoon water
Pecan halves (to garnish)

Melt the butter, add the sugar, and cook until the color deepens. Add the milk and bring to the boil. Blend the cornstarch with about 1 tablespoon water, add it to the mixture, and cook for 1–2 minutes, stirring continuously. Pour into serving dishes or glasses, allow to cool, then decorate with pecan halves. Serves 4.

Honeycomb Mold

2 cups milk
1 tablespoon unflavored
  gelatin
3 tablespoons honey

2 eggs, separated
½ teaspoon vanilla extract
Golden Carrot Cookies*

Scald the milk in the top of a double boiler. Off the heat, slowly sprinkle in the gelatin and stir in the honey. Beat the egg yolks lightly, then pour 3–4 tablespoons of the hot milk over them. Stir, and pour back into the rest of the milk. Place the double boiler over moderate heat and cook very gently, stirring constantly, until the mixture thickens; take care it does not curdle. Add the vanilla extract, then pour into a warmed bowl. Beat the egg whites stiffly and fold in. Turn the mixture gently into a greased 3-cup decorative mold and leave to set. Unmold to serve. The dessert will have a jellied layer on top and a spongy one below. Serve with Golden Carrot Cookies.* Serves 4.

Strawberry Shortcake

2 cups all-purpose flour
2½ teaspoons baking powder
¼ cup butter
2 tablespoons brown sugar
1 egg, beaten

Milk (if needed)
2 cups fresh strawberries
Honey
½–¾ cup heavy cream

Preheat oven to 425° F.

Sift flour and baking powder into a bowl. Cut in the butter and add the brown sugar. Mix in the egg and a little milk if necessary until a stiff dough is obtained. Roll out 1 inch thick. Cut into rounds 3 inches in diameter, and place about 1½ inches apart on a greased cookie sheet. Bake in the hot oven for 7–10 minutes until well risen and browned.

Meanwhile, mash the strawberries and sweeten to taste with honey. In a separate bowl, beat the cream until stiff.

When the shortcakes are done, split in half while still hot and sandwich them together with crushed strawberries. Place more strawberries plus the whipped cream on top. Serves 6.

Strawberry Ice Pudding

1¼ cups thick custard	Whipped cream (to garnish)
2 tablespoons clear honey	Whole strawberries (to
2½ cups crushed fresh	garnish)
strawberries	Pecan halves (to garnish)
1¼ cups heavy cream	

Add the custard and honey to the crushed strawberries. Beat the cream until stiff and fold it into the strawberry mixture.

Put into a container and fast-freeze, stirring from time to time. When set but not completely hard, press into a 2½-pint round mold or bowl. Put a layer of waxed paper under the lid. Seal the join with freezer tape. Refreeze.

To serve, ease out onto a chilled serving dish and decorate with whipped cream, whole strawberries, and pecan halves. Serves 6.

"Chocolate" Pudding

⅓ cup carob powder	1½ tablespoons clear honey
½ cup boiling water	2½ cups cold water
3 tablespoons cornstarch	3 egg yolks
½ cup dried milk powder	1¼ teaspoons vanilla extract
Pinch of sea salt	

Put the carob powder in a small bowl and stir in the boiling water, pressing out any lumps. Set aside.

Mix the cornstarch and dried milk powder together, add a pinch of salt and 1½ tablespoons honey. Gradually add the cold water and whisk well so that all the ingredients are blended.

Combine the carob and cornstarch mixtures in a double boiler over hot simmering water and cook until the pudding thickens, stirring constantly. Cook for another 10–15 minutes.

Beat the egg yolks and then blend them into the pudding mixture. Cook for 2–4 minutes more.

Remove double boiler from the heat and add the vanilla extract. Pour the mixture into a serving dish and allow to cool. Chill in the refrigerator and serve with whipped cream. Serves 6.

"Chocolate" Mousse

4 eggs
1 teaspoon sunflower oil
½ cup carob powder, sifted
3 tablespoons brown sugar

6 tablespoons dry California
  white wine (optional)
6 tablespoons water

Separate the eggs and beat the yolks. Set aside. Put the oil in a
saucepan and heat it. Add the sifted carob powder, brown sugar,
wine, and water. If the wine is not used, add an additional 6 tablespoons water. Stir until the carob and brown sugar dissolve. Stir
the egg yolks into the carob mixture, and remove pan from the
heat. Beat the egg whites very stiff, until they make peaks. Fold
them into the carob mixture, making sure they are completely
blended. Pour into a serving dish or into 4 individual dishes,
and set aside to cool. Serves 4.

Small "Chocolate" Party Cakes

¾ cup all-purpose flour
Pinch of sea salt
1 teaspoon baking powder
1 tablespoon carob powder
¼ cup butter

¼ cup honey
1 egg
A few drops of vanilla extract
Milk (if needed)

Preheat oven to 375° F.

Sift the flour, salt, baking powder, and carob powder together
and mix well. Beat the butter and honey together until creamy.
Beat the egg and add it slowly to the butter and honey, beating all
the time. Add the flour mixture, vanilla extract, and a little milk,
if needed, to make the mixture a soft dropping consistency.

Put the mixture into greased 3-inch muffin pans, filling only ⅔
full. Bake in the moderate oven for 15–20 minutes until lightly
browned. Cool on wire rack. Makes 10–12 cakes.

NOTE: When cold the cakes can be frosted with 7-minute or
butter frosting using carob instead of cocoa in both instances.

Ice Cream with Hot "Chocolate" Sauce

For the sauce

2 tablespoons butter
2 tablespoons carob powder
1 teaspoon cornstarch
2½ cups water
A few drops of vanilla extract
Honey (if needed)

1 pint vanilla ice cream
4–8 teaspoons chopped nuts
  or slivered almonds (to
  garnish)

For the sauce: Melt the butter in a saucepan and stir in the carob powder. Blend the cornstarch with a little water and add to the mixture. Slowly add the rest of the water, stirring continuously to keep the sauce smooth. Add a few drops of vanilla extract. Taste and add honey to sweeten, if required. Continue to cook for a few more minutes, stirring all the time.

Put the ice cream into individual dishes and pour the hot sauce on top. Decorate with 1–2 teaspoons chopped nuts. Serve at once. Serves 4.

Cheese Sandwich Pies

¾ cup butter
2 cups cream or cottage
  cheese or a mixture of both
2 cups sifted all-purpose flour

¼ teaspoon sea salt
1 cup mincemeat or thick
  preserves (cherry or peach)
1 egg yolk, beaten

Preheat oven to 350° F.

Put the first 4 ingredients into a food processor or blender, and process until cottage cheese is smooth and the ingredients are blended to a soft dough. Roll it out ¼ inch thick on a well-floured surface and cut into 2-inch rounds. Place half the rounds on an ungreased cookie sheet. Place about ½ teaspoon mincemeat (for baby mince pies) or preserves in the center of each round on the sheet. Brush the edges with egg yolk. Fit the remaining rounds on top, pressing the edges to seal. Brush tops with egg yolk. Bake for about 20 minutes. Cool on the sheet. Makes about 42 pies.

Maple Syrup Chiffon Pie

1 tablespoon gelatin	⅛ teaspoon sea salt
2 tablespoons cold water	2 eggs, separated
½ cup milk	1½ cups whipping cream
½ cup pure maple syrup, plus	1½ teaspoons vanilla extract
1–2 teaspoons for topping	1 (9-inch) baked pastry shell

Soften the gelatin in the water. Warm the milk, ½ cup maple syrup, and salt in the top of a double boiler over simmering water. Beat the egg yolks lightly, and stir them into the warmed milk mixture. Stir constantly until the custard thickens. Add the softened gelatin, and stir until dissolved. Turn into a chilled bowl. Cool. Meanwhile beat the egg whites until stiff but not dry. Separately, whip half the cream with the vanilla until it holds soft peaks. Set the remaining cream aside for topping. Fold the whipped cream into the cooled maple custard. Then fold in the beaten whites. Turn the filling into the pastry shell evenly. Sweeten the reserved cream with 1–2 teaspoons maple syrup and whip until stiff. Swirl on the pie just before serving. Serves 6–8.

Bread and Butter Pudding

4 slices whole wheat bread	3 eggs, beaten
2 tablespoons butter	⅓ cup pure maple syrup
⅓ cup lightly packed brown	1 teaspoon vanilla extract
sugar	Dash of sea salt
½ teaspoon ground cinnamon	2½ cups milk, scalded
⅓ cup raisins	

Preheat oven to 350° F.

Grease a 1½-quart casserole. Lightly toast the whole wheat bread and spread with the butter. Sprinkle the brown sugar, then the cinnamon, over each slice. Sandwich 2 slices together, then the other two, and cut each sandwich into 4 rectangles making 8 in all. Place these in 1 layer in the casserole and sprinkle with the raisins.

Put the beaten eggs, maple syrup, vanilla extract, and salt in a blender or food processor and blend well. Gradually stir this mixture into the scalded milk and then pour over the toast in the casserole. Place casserole in a pan that contains 1 inch of very hot water. Bake in the preheated oven for 60–70 minutes or until a knife inserted into the pudding comes out clean. Serve warm. Serves 6–8.

Spicy Cinnamon Pudding

4 cups milk	1 teaspoon salt
⅔ cup blackstrap molasses	¾ teaspoon ground cinnamon
⅓ cup honey	¾ teaspoon ground allspice
⅔ cup yellow cornmeal	¼ cup butter

Preheat oven to 300° F.

Grease a 2-quart casserole. Put 3 cups of the milk in a pan with the molasses and honey and heat gently. Meanwhile combine the cornmeal, salt, and spices, then gradually stir this mixture into the hot sweet milk. Add the butter. Cook slowly over a low heat stirring constantly until the mixture thickens—about 10 minutes. Pour into the casserole. Pour the remaining cup of milk over the pudding. Bake in the preheated oven for 3 hours. Serve with whipped cream or vanilla ice cream. Serves 8.

Aromatic Fruit Salad

¾ teaspoon clear honey	4 dates, pitted
Pinch of ground allspice	4 fresh peaches, peeled and
1¼ tablespoons water	pitted
24–30 grapes	⅓ cup unsweetened apple
1 medium eating apple	juice
8 dried apricots	Slivered almonds (to garnish)

Simmer honey and allspice in the water. Cool. Halve grapes and remove seeds. Core and chop apple, including skin. Chop dried apricots and dates. Slice peaches. Put all the fruit, allspice-honey mixture, and apple juice in a bowl and leave to soak until the apricots soften. More apple juice can be added if the apricots take up too much of the liquid. Sprinkle with slivered almonds before serving. Serves 4.

16
Snacks

Beef and Mushroom Patties

1 pound freshly ground beef
1 medium onion, finely chopped
½ cup fine hominy grits
1 cup chopped mushrooms
1 (8-ounce) can peeled tomatoes
1 clove garlic, minced
½ teaspoon prepared mustard

¾ teaspoon Worcestershire sauce
Pinch of dried mixed herbs (Provençal blend)
Sea salt
Freshly ground pepper
1 pound plain piecrust
2 tablespoons butter
Milk

Preheat oven to 425° F.

Mix the beef, onion, hominy, and mushrooms together. Drain the tomatoes and combine them with the garlic, mustard, Worcestershire sauce, herbs, salt, and pepper. Mix everything together well.

Roll out the piecrust about ¼ inch thick on a floured surface and cut it into rounds about 6 inches in diameter by placing a small plate on the rolled-out dough and cutting around it. Place the meat mixture on ½ of each pastry round, leaving the edge bare. Dot with butter. Fold the second half of the pastry over the filling and press the edges of the pastry together to seal. Brush the tops of the patties with milk, prick with a fork, and bake in the

preheated oven for 10 minutes, then reduce the heat to 350° F.
Bake for another 50 minutes, until nicely browned. Serves 4–6.

NOTE: Alternatively, the meat mixture can be placed in the center of the pastry rounds. In this case, dampen the edges and join them together at the top, making an upstanding frill.

Steak Tartare

6 ounces raw ground round steak	Sea salt
1 small onion, finely chopped	Freshly ground pepper
1 tablespoon French mustard	2 eggs
¾ teaspoon paprika	Chopped fresh parsley (to garnish)
Dash of Tabasco	

Combine the beef, onion, mustard, paprika, and Tabasco. Add the salt and pepper. Shape the mixture into 2 patties, making a well in the center of each. Break an egg into each well and garnish with chopped parsley. Serve with slices of buttered pumpernickel. Serves 2.

Spicy Snackburgers

2 hamburger buns	Dash of Tabasco
1 clove garlic, cut in half	Sea salt
6–8 ounces raw, finely ground lean beef	Freshly ground pepper
1 small onion, minced	Tomato slices (to garnish)
2 tablespoons Worcestershire sauce	Cucumber slices (to garnish)

Split buns in half and toast them. Rub the cut sides of the garlic clove over the toasted side of the buns. Combine the ground beef, onion, and Worcestershire sauce. Season with Tabasco, salt, and pepper. Spread the mixture on the garlicky buns and top with slices of tomato and cucumber. Serves 2.

Cottage Delight

½ cup cottage cheese
1½ teaspoons drained bottled
   horseradish
Salt
Freshly ground pepper

1 fresh peach
8 white grapes
Lettuce leaves
6 pitted ripe olives

Mash the cottage cheese and stir in the drained horseradish. Season with salt and freshly ground pepper. Cut the peach into slices, discarding the pit. Halve the grapes and take out the seeds. Place 2 lettuce leaves on a plate, arrange the peach slices in a circle, and pile the cottage cheese mixture in the middle, topped with the halved grapes and olives. Serves 1–2.

Cream Cheese and Date Filled Biscuits

¼ cup all-purpose flour
4 teaspoons baking powder
Sea salt
¾ cup whole wheat flour
¼ cup butter, plus butter for
   spreading

Milk
¼ cup finely chopped pitted
   dates
4 ounces cream cheese
Freshly ground pepper

Preheat oven to 450° F.

Sift the all-purpose flour, baking powder, and a pinch of salt into a large bowl. Stir in the whole wheat flour. Cut in the ¼ cup butter and add enough milk to make a soft manageable dough.

Knead the dough lightly and roll out on a floured surface to a 6-inch round. Divide into 6 pieces, and shape each into a round ¾ inch thick. Place the rounds about 1½ inches apart on a greased cookie sheet. Brush the tops of the rounds with milk and bake for about 15 minutes until well risen and browned. Remove from baking sheet and cool on a rack.

Meanwhile, mix the finely chopped dates into the cream cheese and season.

Split the biscuits and spread with butter. Fill generously with the date-cheese spread. Replace the tops and serve. Serves 6.

Creamy Mushroom Aspic

1 (15-ounce) can jellied
consommé, chilled
2½ teaspoons gelatin
2¼ cups finely chopped
mushrooms, plus 2–3
whole mushrooms (to
garnish)

4 ounces cream cheese
Sea salt
Freshly ground pepper
Chopped chives (to garnish)
1¼ cups liquid aspic

Warm 3 tablespoons of the consommé until liquid, add the gelatin, and stir over very gentle heat until the gelatin is dissolved.

Put the 2¼ cups finely chopped mushrooms in a food processor or blender; add the gelatin mixture, remaining consommé, and cream cheese. Add a little salt and pepper, and blend until smooth. Pour into 4 individual molds or custard cups and refrigerate until set.

Slice the reserved whole mushrooms thinly and arrange them on the molds with the chopped chives. Spoon the liquid aspic on top. Chill until the aspic is set, and serve with brown bread and butter. Serves 4.

Spinach Crêpe Stack

2½ pounds fresh spinach
6 (6½-inch) crêpes

¼ cup heavy cream
Chopped chives

For the sauce

3 tablespoons butter
6 tablespoons flour
1 cup milk
1 egg
Sea salt

Freshly ground pepper
1 clove garlic
½ cup cottage cheese
2 ounces cream cheese

Preheat oven to 375° F.

Wash the spinach and cook in 2 inches of water, quickly for 5–6 minutes. Drain thoroughly and put aside. Do not chop.

For the sauce: Melt the butter in a saucepan and stir in the flour; add the milk, stirring constantly, until the sauce is smooth and comes to a boil. It will be very thick. Beat the egg well, then beat it into the sauce. Season the mixture with salt and freshly ground pepper. Remove from the heat.

Mince the clove of garlic. Combine it with the cottage cheese and cream cheese. Put the mixture in a food processor or blender and blend to a smooth paste. Add salt and pepper. Stir the cheese mixture into the sauce. It will be very thick indeed now.

Take a deep round baking dish a little bigger than the crêpes. Grease it with a little butter. Lay a crêpe flat in the bottom of the buttered dish. Spread some spinach over it and spread a layer of the cheese and filling mixture on top of this. Repeat these layers until the dish is filled up. Finish with a crêpe spread with cheese mixture only. Pour the heavy cream over the lot and sprinkle with the chopped chives. Bake for 45–50 minutes. Cut the crêpe stack into wedges in the dish before lifting out each helping. Serves 4.

Barbecued Spareribs

2½ tablespoons sunflower oil
¾ cup minced onion
1 tablespoon beef bouillon granules
¼ cup honey
⅔ cup hot water
1 clove garlic, minced

5 teaspoons chili powder
¼ teaspoon ground ginger
2½ tablespoons tomato paste
¼ cup white vinegar
2 pounds spareribs (lamb or beef)

Preheat oven to 375° F.

Put the oil in a saucepan and add the onion. Cook gently until tender but do not brown. Meanwhile dissolve the bouillon granules and honey in the hot water. Add the garlic, chili powder, and ginger to the onions. Stirring all the time, add the tomato paste, the vinegar, and the bouillon granules mixture. Simmer gently for about 10 minutes.

Put the spareribs in 1 layer in a roasting pan and spoon a little of the sauce over them. Roast in the moderate oven for 30 minutes. Pour off the excess fat and spoon the remaining sauce over the ribs. Roast for another hour at the same temperature. Serves 4.

Stanley's Italian Sausage

1 pound boned dark chicken meat	Vegetable oil for cooking
1 teaspoon sea salt	
1 teaspoon fennel seeds, crushed	
1 teaspoon crushed chili (if you use whole chili peppers and remove the seeds before crushing them they are not so hot)	

Remove the skin and fat from the chicken meat and grind them to a paste in a food processor using the chopper blade. Set aside. Chop the meat in the food processor, grinding it in short bursts for about 10 seconds, using the chopper blade.

Mix the paste and chopped meat and all the spices together well. Place in a bowl and cover with plastic. Make patties from this mixture as required. It will keep for about a week in the refrigerator.

To cook, heat a little vegetable oil in a skillet and cook the patties slowly, about 5 minutes on each side. Drain and serve immediately. Serves 4.

Skewered Cream Cheese and Chicken

4 ounces cream cheese	Dry white vermouth
Sea salt	4 ounces paper-thin slices cold roast chicken
Freshly ground pepper	

Put the cream cheese in a bowl. Season with salt and pepper. Add as much dry white vermouth as the cheese will take without becoming too thin to spread.

Spread the mixture on the chicken slices, roll up and secure with poultry skewers or wooden picks. Chill in the refrigerator for at least an hour. To serve, cut into bite-size pieces and impale on wooden picks. Serves 4.

Chicken Boats

1 stale loaf French bread
2 tablespoons butter
¼ cup all-purpose flour
⅔–1¼ cups milk
Scant 1 cup chopped cold
  chicken

¼ cup cooked small button
  mushrooms
Sea salt
Freshly ground pepper
Chopped fresh mixed herbs as
  available

Preheat oven to 375° F.

Split the loaf in half lengthwise and cut across into 2 or 4 portions. Scoop out the center of each portion.

Melt the butter in a pan. Mix in the flour, and slowly add ½ cup milk. Cook gently until the sauce thickens, stirring constantly. Add more milk as necessary to maintain a thick, creamy consistency. Add the chopped chicken and the mushrooms to the mixture, season with salt, freshly ground pepper, and mixed herbs. The mixture should be quite thick.

Fill the bread portions with the chicken mixture, wrap each in foil, and bake in the moderate oven for 20–30 minutes. Serves 2–4.

Sweet-sour Chicken Drumsticks

4 chicken drumsticks
Melted butter
Sea salt
Freshly ground pepper

4 small onions
¼ cup warmed honey
4–8 teaspoons thyme vinegar
Paprika

Preheat oven to 425° F.

Wipe the drumsticks and brush with melted butter. Season with salt and pepper. Slice the onions and dip the slices in the honey. Cut 4 pieces of aluminum foil large enough to cover each drumstick completely. Arrange dipped onion slices overlapping on each piece of foil and sprinkle with the vinegar. Place the chicken on top. Fold up foil to cover the chicken, forming a small parcel. Bake in the hot oven for 30–45 minutes. Serve chicken with onion on top, sprinkled with paprika. Serves 4.

Chicken Loaf

1 medium onion
1 tablespoon butter
2 cups soft bread crumbs
1 cup diced cooked carrots
2 tablespoons chopped
  nutmeats
1 cup cooked green peas

1 teaspoon dried sage
Sea salt
Freshly ground pepper
2 cups chopped skinned
  cooked chicken
2 eggs, separated

Preheat oven to 350° F.

Chop the onion and brown it lightly in the butter, in a large pan. Add the bread crumbs, carrots, nutmeats, peas, and seasonings. Mix well with a large spoon, then add the chicken. Beat the egg yolks lightly and mix them in. Beat the egg whites stiffly and fold in evenly.

Turn into a well-greased loaf pan. Bake for 1½ hours. Leave to stand for 5 minutes. Serve hot from the pan. Serves 4.

Turkey Sesame Balls

1 cup finely chopped cooked
  turkey
1 tablespoon minced onion
1 small clove garlic, minced
  (optional)
1 teaspoon curry powder

¼ teaspoon paprika
¼ teaspoon turmeric
3 tablespoons mayonnaise
⅓ cup sesame seeds
Parsley sprigs (to garnish)

Preheat oven to 350° F.

Combine the cooked turkey, minced onion, garlic, curry powder, paprika, and turmeric in a small bowl and mix well. Gradually add the mayonnaise and mix until thoroughly blended. Form the mixture into small balls, using about 1 teaspoonful for each. Cover and chill thoroughly in the refrigerator.

Meanwhile toast the sesame seeds in the oven until golden brown, about 5 to 10 minutes.

Roll the chilled turkey balls in the toasted sesame seeds. Place on a serving dish and garnish with sprigs of fresh parsley. Keep refrigerated until ready to serve. Makes about 24 balls.

Crispy Golden Eggs

5 eggs
Sea salt
Freshly ground pepper
1 cup dry bread crumbs
¼ teaspoon dried thyme

¼ teaspoon dried oregano
¼ teaspoon dried sage
¼ teaspoon dried marjoram
Flour
Oil for deep frying

Hard-cook 4 of the eggs. Break the other egg into a bowl and beat it with a little salt and pepper.

Finely crush the bread crumbs, adding the dried herbs.

When the hard-cooked eggs are cold, sprinkle them with flour, dip them in the raw egg, and then roll them in the bread crumb mixture. Fry the eggs quickly in deep hot oil and serve with sweet pickle and slices of cucumber. Serves 2.

Curried Poached Eggs

1 small onion
¼ cup butter
1 tablespoon curry powder
¾ teaspoon Worcestershire
  sauce

2 cups tomato juice
4 eggs
2 slices buttered whole wheat
  toast

Finely chop the onion and sauté it in the butter. Add the curry powder and Worcestershire sauce, and cook quickly, stirring constantly, for 2–3 minutes. Take off the heat, but keep warm.

Put the tomato juice in a saucepan and heat to simmering point. Poach the eggs in the tomato juice. When they are done, put them on the whole wheat toast and pour the onion-curry sauce over them. Serve immediately. Serves 2.

Poached Eggs with Spinach

1 pound leaf spinach
Sea salt
2 large eggs

4 teaspoons chilled butter,
  flaked
Freshly ground pepper

Carefully wash and drain the spinach. Put 2 inches of water in a large pan and bring to the boil, add a little salt and the spinach. Cook quickly for 5–6 minutes or until tender but not mushy.

Meanwhile, poach the eggs in an egg poacher or pan of water. Drain the spinach well and place on 2 hot plates. Top each helping of spinach with flaked butter and a poached egg sprinkled with salt and freshly ground pepper. For a more substantial meal, allow 2 eggs per person. Serves 2.

Tuna-stuffed Eggs

6 eggs
2 tablespoons mayonnaise
½ teaspoon cider vinegar
4 scallions, finely chopped
⅓ cup mashed drained tuna
   fish

Sea salt
Freshly ground pepper
Fresh chopped chives or
   parsley (to garnish)

Hard-cook the eggs. Crack and drop them into cold water. When cold, remove their shells. Cut the eggs in half lengthwise, and carefully take out the yolks. Reserve the white halves.

Combine the yolks with the mayonnaise, cider vinegar, chopped scallions, and mashed tuna fish. Season with salt and pepper and blend until smooth.

Refill the egg whites with the mixture and sprinkle chopped fresh chives or parsley on top. Makes 12 halves.

Scotch Eggs

1 (1¾-ounce) can anchovy
   fillets
2½ tablespoons milk
6 hard-cooked eggs
Sea salt
Freshly ground pepper
A few drops of Worcestershire
   sauce

Whole wheat flour
1 egg, beaten
¼ cup toasted, fine, whole
   wheat bread crumbs
Oil for deep frying

Drain the oil from the anchovy fillets and soak them in the milk for 10 minutes. Meanwhile, cut the hard-cooked eggs in half and scoop out the yolks.

Take the anchovy fillets out of the milk. Discard the milk and mash them with the egg yolks. Add salt and pepper and a few drops of Worcestershire sauce. Stuff the mixture into the egg whites and stick the 2 halves together again.

Coat the eggs in flour, beaten egg, and the toasted fine whole wheat bread crumbs. Put in the refrigerator for 30 minutes, then deep fry the eggs in very hot oil until golden brown. Drain and serve. Serves 6.

Fish Ribbon Loaf

¼ cup butter
¼ cup minced shallots or mild onion
¼ cup pastry flour
1 teaspoon dried dill
1½ cups light cream or half-and-half

1½ pounds white fish fillets, skinned and cut up
3 eggs, beaten
Sea salt
White pepper
1 cup canned or cooked salmon, flaked

Preheat oven to 350° F.

Melt the butter in a large skillet over low heat, add the shallots, and stir until they soften. Mix in the flour and stir for about 1 minute. Add the dill and cream, and continue stirring until the sauce reaches the boiling point. As soon as it thickens, stir in the pieces of fish and the eggs. Remove from the heat. Season well.

Put half the mixture in a food processor or blender and process until smooth. Spread it in an even layer in a greased 8½ × 4½ × 3-inch loaf pan. Cool slightly.

Spread the flaked salmon over the mixture in the pan. Process the remaining white fish mixture in the processor or blender, and spread it over the salmon.

Place the pan in a baking pan, and add 1½ inches boiling water to the baking pan. Bake for 30 minutes. Cool in the loaf pan on a rack, then chill until needed. Serve in squares or slices with mayonnaise. Serves 6.

Cold Rolled Flounder Fillets

4 flounder fillets (about 6
  ounces each), skinned
Butter for greasing
About 1 cup dry California
  white wine
1 sprig fresh or 1 teaspoon
  dried thyme

1 bay leaf
Freshly ground pepper
Scrambled Eggs Petrovitch*
4 small rounds fried bread

Preheat oven to 350° F.

Trim the fillets neatly. Cut a strip of waxed paper the same
width as each fillet and long enough to roll up into a solid cigar-
sized tube. Roll up the strips. Place one across the tail end of
each fillet and roll up the fillet around it. Secure with wooden
toothpicks. Stand the fillets on end in a well-buttered shallow
baking dish, and pour enough wine around them to come halfway
up their sides. Add the herbs and season with pepper. Bake for
about 10 minutes, basting twice. Cool.

Drain the fillets, remove the toothpicks, and take out the paper
rolls carefully without breaking the fillets open. Fill the small
spaces left by the rolls with Scrambled Eggs Petrovitch.* Serve on
small rounds of fried bread. Serves 4.

NOTE: Pompano, sole, or whiting fillets can be used. As alternative fillings, try Cheesy Scrambled Eggs* or Tuna Mousse.*

Salmon Layers

3 tablespoons butter
2 cups fresh whole wheat
  bread crumbs
1 (8-ounce) can red salmon,
  drained
¼ cup light cream
1½ teaspoons dry white wine
¾ cup cottage cheese

Sea salt
Freshly ground pepper
Cucumber slices (to garnish)
2 tomatoes, sliced (to
  garnish)
2 raw mushrooms, sliced (to
  garnish)

Melt the butter in a skillet and fry bread crumbs until browned; set aside to cool.

Mash the salmon well with the cream and add the wine. Place ⅔ of the bread crumbs in a shallow dish. Mash the cottage cheese and spread it over the bread crumbs. Season with salt and pepper. Place the salmon mixture on top and sprinkle the remainder of the bread crumbs over the salmon. Decorate with the cucumber, tomatoes, and mushrooms. Serves 4.

Sardine Pâté

1 (4⅜-ounce) can sardines in oil
1 small onion
Small bunch chives or green onions
¼ cup butter
1 cup cottage cheese
5 teaspoons dry white wine
1 teaspoon tomato paste
Sea salt
Freshly ground pepper
Thin cucumber slices (to garnish)
Watercress sprigs (to garnish)

Chop the sardines, discarding the bigger bones. Mince the onion. Chop the chives or green onions. Cut the butter into small pieces. Put all these ingredients into a food processor or blender and add the cheese, wine, tomato paste, and salt and pepper. Blend until thoroughly mixed into a smooth paste.

Turn into a bowl and garnish with thin slices of cucumber and sprigs of watercress. Refrigerate until needed. Serves 6.

Tuna Mousse

2 (7-ounce) cans tuna in oil
2 tablespoons chopped pitted ripe olives
2 cloves garlic
4 teaspoons olive oil or oil from tuna can
½ cup heavy cream
A few drops of white vinegar
Pinch of curry powder
Pinch of ground allspice

Drain the tuna, but reserve the oil if you are not using olive oil. Mix the fish and olives. Crush the garlic in a garlic crusher and mix the juice into the oil. Put all the ingredients in a food processor or blender, and process until smooth. Add extra oil to make a softer mousse or to make it into a dip if desired. Serves 6.

Tuna and Corn Pie

8 ounces plain pastry dough
3 tablespoons butter
6 tablespoons whole wheat
  flour
1¼ cups milk
1 (7-ounce) can whole corn,
  drained
2 eggs, beaten
1 (7-ounce) can water-packed
  tuna, drained and flaked

1¼ tablespoons tomato paste
¾ teaspoon Worcestershire
  sauce
Sea salt
Freshly ground pepper
2 tomatoes, sliced
Melted butter

Preheat oven to 400° F.

Roll the pastry out into a 12-inch circle. Grease a 9-inch pie plate, then line it with the pastry, ensuring that it does not crack.

Melt the butter in a saucepan and stir in the flour. Gradually add the milk, stirring constantly over a gentle heat until the sauce is smooth. When the sauce reaches boiling point, add the corn. Mix in the eggs and stir in the flaked tuna. Add the tomato paste, Worcestershire sauce, salt, and freshly ground pepper to taste.

Spread the mixture on the pastry in the pie plate, arrange sliced tomatoes on top, and brush the surface with melted butter. Put the pie into the hot oven for 10 minutes, then reduce the heat to 350° F. and continue baking for another 30 minutes. Cool the pie in the pie plate. This pie freezes well. Serves 4–6.

Cream Cheese and Walnut Sandwiches

Cayenne
4 ounces cream cheese
½ cup walnuts, finely
  chopped or coarsely ground

Buttered brown bread
Watercress sprigs (to garnish)

Mix cayenne to taste into the cream cheese. Add the walnuts. Mix well. Spread the mixture on slices of buttered brown bread and make into sandwiches. Garnish with watercress. Serves 2–4.

French Sardine Sandwich

1 small loaf French bread
1 (4⅜-ounce) can sardines in oil

Mayonnaise

Preheat broiler.

Cut the French bread into 2 pieces, each about 6 inches long, and split them lengthwise. Toast the bread lightly on the crust side only (not the cut side). Now put the toasted bread, cut side up, in the broiler pan. Place the sardines on the bread and spoon the sardine oil over both the bread and fish so that the bread is nicely saturated. Broil for 3–5 minutes about 6 inches from the source of heat until nicely browned. Remove and spread thickly with mayonnaise. Serve immediately. Serves 2.

NOTE: If you are very hungry you may use 2 cans of sardines!

Piquant Cheese Open Sandwich

Butter
4 Pumpernickel slices
4–6 ripe olives, pitted
4 ounces cream cheese
A few drops of Worcestershire sauce

Freshly ground pepper
2 tablespoons light cream or as needed
Chopped fresh parsley (to garnish)

Lightly butter the pumpernickel. Mash the pitted olives and combine them with the cream cheese. Add a few drops of Worcestershire sauce, the freshly ground pepper, and enough cream to make a spreadable mixture. Spread on the slices of pumpernickel and garnish with chopped parsley. Serves 2.

Bumper Decker Sandwiches

2 hard-cooked eggs
2½ tablespoons thick
  mayonnaise
12 slices whole wheat bread
½ cup butter
½ cup mashed tuna fish
¾ cup finely sliced cucumber

Sea salt
Freshly ground pepper
½ cup cottage cheese
¾ cup sliced canned red
  pimiento
Parsley sprigs (to garnish)

Chop the eggs and mix to a paste with the mayonnaise (do this in a food processor or blender).

Spread the sliced bread with butter. Place 3 slices, butter side up, on a flat surface. Spread each slice with mashed tuna fish, top with slices of cucumber, and season lightly. Top each slice with another slice of buttered bread (buttered side up). Season the cheese and spread it on the bread. Cover with the pimiento slices. Top each of these sandwiches with another slice of bread, buttered side up, spread with the hard-cooked egg, mayonnaise, and seasoning. Finish with remaining slices of bread, this time buttered side down. Press lightly, wrap each sandwich in foil, and refrigerate for about 45 minutes. Cut each decker into 2 triangles. Serve garnished with parsley. Serves 6.

Cream Cheese Sandwiches

4 ounces cream cheese
1¼ teaspoons minced
  horseradish
¾ teaspoon Worcestershire
  sauce
Sea salt

Freshly ground pepper
About 1 tablespoon light
  cream
1 tablespoon chopped fresh
  parsley
Whole wheat bread

Put the cream cheese in a bowl, beat in the horseradish, Worcestershire sauce, salt, and freshly ground pepper. Add enough cream to make a good spreading consistency. Add the chopped parsley. Sandwich between thin slices of whole wheat bread. (This spread is also good on whole wheat crackers.) Serves 2–4.

Salad Niçoise

For the salad

1 head lettuce
1 (7-ounce) can water-packed
    tuna
2 hard-cooked eggs
10 pitted ripe olives
6 anchovy fillets
½ sweet red bell pepper,
    seeded and chopped

8 radishes, cut in rosettes
A few capers
A small piece of chopped
    fennel bulb
Minced chives

For the French dressing

1 clove garlic, finely chopped
2 tablespoons white wine
    vinegar
5 tablespoons olive oil

Pinch of sea salt
Freshly ground pepper
½ teaspoon clear honey

For the salad: Wash the lettuce, dry, and cut into quarters. Arrange in the salad bowl. Drain the tuna, divide into pieces, and add it to the lettuce together with slices of hard-cooked egg. Add the rest of the ingredients to make a decorative salad.

For the dressing: Prepare a French dressing with the ingredients above and toss with the salad just before serving. Serves 2–4.

Cauliflower, Tuna, and Cottage Cheese Salad

1 tart eating apple (Granny
    Smith, Cox's)
2 tablespoons cider vinegar
1 small head cauliflower
1 (7-ounce) can tuna in oil
½ cup cottage cheese
1 small clove garlic, minced
1 teaspoon prepared mustard

1½ tablespoons chopped
    chives
Sea salt
Freshly ground pepper
2–3 lettuce leaves or
    watercress sprigs (to
    garnish)

Peel and core the apple and cut or chop into small pieces. In a bowl toss apple pieces in the cider vinegar to coat. Break the cauliflower into small florets. Drain the oil from the tuna and flake the fish into a bowl. Mix together the cottage cheese, garlic, mustard, and chopped chives in a separate bowl. Season with salt and pepper. Fold in the chopped apple, cauliflower florets, and tuna.

Serve the salad garnished with lettuce or watercress and accompanied by slices of whole wheat bread. Serves 4.

Cream of Cauliflower and Almond Soup

1 head cauliflower	Sea salt
4⅓ cups milk	Freshly ground pepper
1 tablespoon chicken bouillon granules	4–6 tablespoons heavy cream
¼ cup ground almonds	¼ cup slivered toasted almonds (to garnish)

Wash the cauliflower and break into florets. Bring to the boil, 2 cups of the milk to which the bouillon granules have been added. Cook the cauliflower gently in the boiling milk for about 10 minutes. Process cauliflower and cooking liquid in a food processor or blender and return the mixture to the saucepan; add the ground almonds and enough milk to make the soup a creamy consistency. Reheat, stirring constantly. Season with salt and freshly ground pepper.

Serve with a spoonful of cream ladled into the center of each bowl of soup and garnish with the toasted slivered almonds. Serves 4–6.

Cream of Watercress Soup

2 small onions	1 tablespoon chicken bouillon granules
2 bunches watercress	
3 tablespoons butter	Sea salt
¼ cup flour	Freshly ground pepper
5 cups milk	4–6 teaspoons heavy cream

Mince the onions. Reserve ½ bunch of watercress on one side. Chop the other 1½ bunches. Melt the butter in a saucepan and gently fry the onions and watercress until the onions are clear. Add the flour and mix into a paste. Gradually add the milk, stirring constantly. Add the bouillon granules. Bring the soup to the boil and simmer for about 10 minutes. Season with salt and pepper. Sieve or process the soup in a food processor or blender and return it to the saucepan. Heat through.

Chop the remaining ½ bunch of watercress coarsely and add it to the soup just before serving. Add a teaspoon of heavy cream to each helping. Serves 4–6.

Cream of Mushroom Soup

1 small onion	Scant 2 cups milk
1 small clove garlic	Sea salt
¼–⅓ cup butter	Freshly ground pepper
3 cups finely chopped	¼ cup heavy cream
mushrooms	4 teaspoons chopped fresh
¼ cup all-purpose flour	parsley (to garnish)

Mince the onion and garlic. Heat the butter in a saucepan and when it has melted, add the onion and garlic. Cook them gently until the onion is clear. Do not brown. Add a quarter of the mushrooms, put a lid on the pan, and cook gently for 2–4 minutes. Stir in the flour and gradually add the milk, stirring constantly. When half the milk has been added, put in the rest of the mushrooms. Cook for 5 minutes and then add the rest of the milk.

Cook gently for another 15–20 minutes, stirring regularly. Season with salt and pepper.

Serve with a spoonful of cream floating on the top of each bowl of soup. Garnish with the chopped parsley and some coarsely ground pepper. Serves 4.

17

Beverages

Nonalcoholic

Apple and Cucumber Shake

2 eating apples
⅓ cucumber

2½ tablespoons cider vinegar
2 cups cold water

Peel and core the apples. Cut into pieces and put in a blender or food processor. Cut a few slices of cucumber and set aside. Peel the rest of the cucumber and add to the blender together with the cider vinegar and water. Blend until smooth. Add more water to ensure a pouring consistency if necessary. Serve chilled in tall glasses. Decorate with a slice of cucumber from those set aside. Serves 2.

Apple Ginger Fizz

Unsweetened apple juice
Ground ginger
Carbonated water

Unpeeled apple slices (to garnish)

Fill each glass half full of unsweetened apple juice. Sprinkle on ground ginger to taste. Fill rest of glass with carbonated water. Stir well and decorate with a slice of unpeeled apple.

Hot Mulled Apple Juice

5 cups unsweetened apple
   juice
1 (2½-inch) piece cinnamon
   stick

5 whole cloves

Put the juice, cinnamon, and cloves in a pan and bring to the boil. Reduce the heat and simmer the mixture for about 20 minutes. Strain and serve hot in mugs. Serves 4–6.

Minty Apple Cup

2½ cups cider
1¼ cups mint tea
Ice cubes

Fresh mint sprigs (to garnish)
Cucumber slices (to garnish)

Mix cider and tea together. Add lots of ice cubes, sprigs of fresh mint, and slices of cucumber. If you can eat citrus fruits, this is delicious with slices of fresh lemon. Serves 4.

Apricot Shake

2 cups pitted fresh apricots
   (or dried apricots soaked
   overnight)

4 cups milk
½ cup clear honey

Slice the apricots and place in a blender with 1 cup of the milk and the honey. Blend, then add the remaining milk and blend again. Serve chilled. Serves 4–6.

"Chocolate" Eggnog

1 tablespoon clear honey
2 cups milk

4 teaspoons carob powder
1 egg, beaten

Dissolve the honey in a little of the milk, then beat or blend together all the ingredients. Serve chilled. Serves 2.

"Chocolate" Milk Shake (1)

2 tablespoons clear honey   6 tablespoons carob powder
2½ cups milk

Melt the honey in a little hot water, then combine it with the milk. Pour in the carob powder and beat well with egg beater. Alternatively, whirl the whole lot in a blender or food processor. Serve chilled in tall glasses. Serves 2–4.

"Chocolate" Milk Shake (2)

1¼ cups milk   1 tablespoon carob powder
1 teaspoon clear honey   ½ teaspoon vanilla extract

Put all ingredients in a food processor or blender and blend until smooth. Serve hot. Serves 1.

"Chocolate" Milk Shake (3)

2 tablespoons carob powder   2 teaspoons clear honey
2 tablespoons sunflower oil   A few drops of vanilla extract
2½ cups milk

Dissolve the carob powder in the oil and add a little milk. Put over a gentle heat for a few minutes to cook the carob. Take the mixture off the heat and blend it with the rest of the milk, honey, and the vanilla extract. This can be served hot or cold. Serves 2.

Grape Punch

1 cup dry white grape juice   2 cups cider
1 dessert pear, peeled and   Mint sprigs (to garnish)
  cored

Put all the ingredients in the blender. When well blended dilute with water to desired strength. Serve chilled decorated with sprigs of mint. Serves 4.

Hot Mulled Pineapple Juice

5 cups unsweetened pineapple juice
1 (2-inch) piece cinnamon stick

3–4 cloves
Pinch of grated nutmeg
Pinch of ground allspice

Pour the juice into a pan and add the cinnamon stick, cloves, and spices. Heat until boiling, then reduce the heat, put a lid on the pan, and simmer the mixture for about 20 minutes. Remove from the heat, take out the cinnamon stick and cloves, and serve hot in mugs. Serves 4.

Nighttime "Chocolate"

1½–2½ teaspoons carob powder
2½ tablespoons water

⅔ cup milk
A few drops of vanilla extract

Put the carob powder in a cup and mix it with the water until a smooth paste is obtained. Put the milk in a saucepan and heat. Just before the milk boils, take it off the heat and pour it onto the carob paste, stirring constantly. Return the mixture to the pan for 2–3 minutes and add a few drops of vanilla extract. Serve hot. Serves 1.

Coffee Nog

1 cup milk
1 egg yolk

1 teaspoon clear honey
A few drops of coffee extract

Mix all the ingredients together in a blender or food processor. Any permitted flavoring of your choice can be substituted for the coffee. Serves 1.

Fresh Currant Drink

Fresh currants (black or red)
Clear honey

Pinch of ground cloves

Wash the currants and pick the berries off the stems. Use equal amounts of berries and water and simmer until soft. Sieve to remove tops and tails. Cool, then blend in a food processor or blender until smooth. Sweeten to taste with honey and add a pinch of ground cloves. Put in a large jug with lots of ice.

Summer Sparkler

Pineapple juice
Ginger ale
Ice cubes made from
   pineapple juice

Candied cherries
Cucumber slices

For each person, fill a tall glass ⅔ full with pineapple juice and flavor to taste with ginger ale. Add pineapple ice cubes, candied cherries, and slices of cucumber.

Pineapple Treat

2 glasses unsweetened
   pineapple juice
2 tart eating apples

Clear honey
Maraschino cherries (to
   garnish)

Put the pineapple juice in a food processor or blender. Peel and core the apples, chop them, and add them to the juice. Blend until smooth. Add honey to taste. Blend again. Serve chilled in tall glasses decorated with maraschino cherries. Serves 2.

Melon Refresher

1 small cantaloupe
Unsweetened pineapple juice

Crushed ice
Fresh mint sprigs (to garnish)

Peel the cantaloupe and discard the seeds. Cut into pieces and process in a blender or food processor with a little of the unsweetened pineapple juice. Put into a large jug with plenty of crushed ice. Thin down the mixture with unsweetened pineapple juice and garnish with sprigs of fresh mint. Serves 2–4.

Pineapple Sour

½ bunch fresh watercress   Ice cubes
1 (19-fluid-ounce) can
  pineapple juice

Cut off most of the stems and add the fresh watercress leaves to a large can of pineapple juice. Mix in a blender or food processor until smooth. This makes a lovely combination of sweet and bitter. Serve over ice. Serves 4.

Sunshine Shake

½ cup canned pineapple juice   Fresh or canned pineapple
1¼ cups ice-cold milk   cubes (to garnish)
Fresh mint sprigs (to garnish)

Mix the pineapple juice and ice-cold milk together and shake or beat until the mixture froths. Pretty up each serving with a sprig of mint and a few cubes of pineapple. Serves 2.

Tiger's Milk

2½ cups milk   1 tablespoon molasses
1¼ tablespoons brewers' yeast
1 (19-fluid-ounce) can
  pineapple juice

Whirl all the ingredients together in a blender or food processor and serve chilled. Serves 2–4.

Hot Vegetable Juice

1 (12½-fluid-ounce) can V8   Sea salt
  juice   Freshly ground pepper
1 clove garlic

Empty vegetable juice into a saucepan and add the clove of garlic sliced into 3–4 pieces. Bring to the boil and simmer for a few minutes. Add salt and pepper to taste. Serve hot. Serves 1–2.

Alcoholic

Everyman's Champagne

White wine, chilled
Carbonated water, chilled

Simply mix ⅓ wine to ⅔ carbonated water. If you like it sweet, try Graves or Sauterne, if you prefer it dry, try Hock or Chablis.

White Wine Cobbler

2 tablespoons clear honey
½ cup carbonated water, chilled

1½ cups California medium-dry white wine, chilled

Mix all the ingredients together. Serves 2.

Apple Julep

2½ cups unsweetened apple juice
1¼ cups unsweetened pineapple juice

⅔ cup dry white wine
⅔ cup carbonated water
Fresh mint sprigs (to garnish)

Mix all the ingredients together. Pour into a large container with plenty of ice and decorate with sprigs of fresh mint. Serves 4.

Ginger Grape Cocktail

1¼ cups dry white wine
1¼ cups white grape juice
1¼ cups carbonated water

1½ teaspoons ground ginger
Ice cubes
Cucumber slices (to garnish)

Mix first 4 ingredients together well. Serve with ice and slices of cucumber. Serves 3–4.

White Wine Punch

1 standard-size bottle dry
   white vermouth
1 standard-size bottle dry
   white wine
2 cups strong tea
1 cup honey syrup
1 quart carbonated water
Cucumber slices (to garnish)

Mix together all the ingredients except the cucumber and refrigerate. Decorate with slices of cucumber, and serve chilled. Serves 8.

White Wine Cup

1 standard-size bottle
   California dry white wine
½ cup dry white vermouth
1 cup carbonated water
Clear honey
Ice cubes
Fresh pineapple, sliced thinly
   (to garnish)
Fresh mint sprigs (to garnish)

Mix wine, vermouth, and carbonated water together. Sweeten with the honey and serve with lots of ice, decorated with the slices of fresh pineapple and sprigs of mint. Serves 4.

Champagne Julep

1 sprig fresh mint
Cucumber slices
Ice cubes
Champagne
1 lump sugar (optional)

Put mint and cucumber into a wineglass with ice and pour champagne over, stirring all the while, then add the sugar. Serves 1.

Mint Champagne

1 teaspoon green crème de menthe
Champagne or dry white sparkling wine

Put 1 teaspoon of crème de menthe in a champagne glass and fill with chilled champagne or white sparkling wine. Serves 1.

Moonlight Fizz

1 egg white
½ cup gin
1¼ teaspoons clear honey

20 drops angostura bitters
Crushed ice
Carbonated water

Beat egg white well. Mix gin, honey, angostura bitters, and crushed ice. Add the egg white and shake well. Strain ⅓ mixture into each cocktail glass and fill up with carbonated water. Serves 2–4.

Fruit Cup

1 pound fruit in season, such
   as peaches, strawberries,
   cherries, or apricots
1 cup clear honey

2–3 pints carbonated water,
   chilled
1 cup gin, chilled

Wash the fruit, take out the pits or seeds. Reserve some for garnish. Slice the rest into a bowl with the honey. Let it stand overnight. When ready to use, pour into the chilled sparkling water. Add 1 cup of gin. Serve decorated with the reserved fruit. Serves 8.

Lager Shandy

Lager
Ginger ale

Crushed ice

Combine equal parts lager and ginger ale. Mix together well, add crushed ice, and serve.

Adonis

2 tablespoons Italian dry
   vermouth
¼ cup Rose's lime juice

2 drops angostura bitters
Ice cubes

Mix ingredients together. Stir briefly. Serves 1.

Strawberry Champagne Punch

2 pounds fresh strawberries
A little clear honey
2 bottles champagne or dry
white sparkling wine

A large cake of ice or ice
cubes

Hull the strawberries and cover them with a little clear honey. Add 1 pint of the champagne and let stand for about 5 hours. Do not refrigerate. Chill the rest of the champagne.

Place the cake of ice or a large quantity of ice cubes in a punch bowl and pour the strawberry mixture over. Add the rest of the champagne, well chilled, and let stand until the liquid becomes a delicate shade of pink. Serve at once. Serves 10–12.

Champagne Fruit Punch

1 fresh pineapple
5 cups California dry white
wine

Melted honey, cooled
1 bottle champagne, chilled

Peel the pineapple and cut into cubes. Marinate in 5 cups white wine for 12 hours in freezer. Add melted honey to taste, plus 1 bottle champagne. Serve chilled. Serves 4–6.

Country Club Cooler

2 measures dry vermouth
1 teaspoon grenadine

Ice cubes
Carbonated water, chilled

Combine dry vermouth and grenadine in a tall glass with ice and fill with chilled carbonated water. Serves 1.

Italian Tonic

Dry white vermouth
Tonic water

Cucumber slice
Ice cubes

Mix dry white vermouth with tonic water, add a slice of cucumber, and lots of ice. Serves 1.

Appendix I

National Migraine Foundation

The National Migraine Foundation was formed in 1971 by a prestigious group of medical professionals as a nonprofit-making organization dedicated to the headache sufferer and his or her family.

The aims of the foundation are:

- to determine the causes of headache and provide treatment as quickly as possible
- to encourage the growth of headache treatment centers throughout the United States
- to educate and promote interest in headaches by physicians and the public (many people currently suffer needlessly due to lack of knowledge about their problem).

The foundation is dependent upon support and donations from its members. A minimum donation of $10 (1983) is required for membership. Members receive a quarterly newsletter prepared for headache sufferers. This publication contains the most recent and up-to-date information about headaches of all types that is currently available locally and on an international level, and provides many interesting and helpful suggestions for headache management.

The National Migraine Foundation will also provide, at a member's request, the names of doctors in his or her area who are members of The American Association for the Study of Headache.

For further information contact: National Migraine Foundation, 5252 North Western Avenue, Chicago, Illinois 60625, Telephone: (312) 878-7715.

Appendix II

Headache Clinics and Other Useful Addresses (as of July 1982)

The American Association for the Study of Headache
5252 North Western Avenue
Chicago, Illinois 60625
Telephone: (312) 878-5558

ARIZONA

Headache Group of the Southwest
1402 North Miller Road, Suite F-5,
Scottsdale, Arizona 85257
Attention: G. Scott Tyler, M.D.
Telephone: (602) 941-5353

Dr. Arnold Friedman Neurological Associates of Tucson
Tucson Medical Park
Tucson, Arizona

CALIFORNIA

Beverly Hills Headache and Pain Medical Group
9400 Brighton Way, Suite 410
Beverly Hills, California 90210
Attention: Gunnar Heuser, M.D., Ph.D.

Pain Treatment Center
Hospital of Scripps Clinic and Foundation
10666 North Torrey Pines Road
La Jolla, California 92037
Attention: Richard A. Sternbach, Ph.D.
Telephone: (714) 455-8898

Valley Multispeciality Pain Center
15216 Vanowen Street, Suite 2D
Van Nuys, California 91405
Attention: Gary W. Jay, M.D.

The New England Center for Headache
40 East Putham Avenue
Cos Cob, Connecticut 06807
Attention: Alan M. Rapoport, M.D.
Telephone: (203) 661-3900

FLORIDA

The Headache Institute
1135 Kane Concourse
Bay Harbor Islands
Miami Beach, Florida 33154
Attention: Larry S. Eisner, M.D.

ILLINOIS

Diamond Headache Clinic, Ltd.
5252 North Western Avenue
Chicago, Illinois 60625
Attention: Seymour Diamond, M.D.
Telephone: (312) 878-5558

KANSAS

Headache Research and Treatment Center
Menninger Foundation
5800 SW 6th Avenue, Building 8
Topeka, Kansas 66601
University of Kansas Medical Center
Department of Medicine
Kansas City, Kansas 66103
Attention: Dewey K. Ziegler, M.D.
Telephone: (913) 588-6985

MASSACHUSETTS

The Headache Research Foundation
Patient Care Division
Professional Office Suite at Faulkner Hospital, Suite 5975
Jamaica Plain, Massachusetts 02130
Attention: Mrs. Liz Heatley (Executive Secretary)
Telephone: (617) 522-6969

MICHIGAN

Michigan Headache and Neurological Institute
3120 Professional Drive
Ann Arbor, Michigan 48104
Attention: Joel Saper, M.D.
Telephone: (313) 973-1155

MISSOURI

Ryan Headache Center
Mercy Doctors Building, Suite 537
621 South New Ballas Road
St. Louis, Missouri 63141
Attention: Robert E. Ryan, Sr., M.D.
Telephone: (314) 872-8778

NEBRASKA

Biofeedback and Headache Clinic
Midlands Medical Center, Suite 333
401 East Gold Coast Road
Papillion, Nebraska 68128
Attention: Jan J. Golnick, M.D.

NEW YORK

Center for Stress and Pain Related Disorders
Columbia-Presbyterian Medical Center
Columbian-Presbyterian South
38–40 East 61st Street
New York, New York 10021
Telephone: (212) 595-3169
Comprehensive Pain Center
New York University Medical Center
530 First Avenue at 32nd Street
New York, New York 10016
Telephone: (212) 340-6622
Facial Pain-TMJ Clinic
Columbia University School of Dental and Oral Surgery
630 West 168th Street
New York, New York 10032

Attention: Joseph Marbach, M.D.
Telephone: (212) 694-4185
Headache Clinic
Mount Sinai Hospital Medical Center
11 East 100th Street
New York, New York 10029
Attention: David Coddon, M.D.
ALSO AT:
1 Gustave Levy Place
New York, New York 10029
Telephone: (212) 650-7691
Headache Unit
Montefiore Hospital
111 East 210th Street
Bronx, New York 10467
Attention: Seymour Solomon, M.D.
Telephone: (212) 920-4636

OHIO

The Cleveland Clinic
9500 Euclid Avenue
Cleveland, Ohio 44106
The Migraine Association of Cincinnati
P. O. Box 29382
Cincinnati, Ohio 45229

TEXAS

Anesthesiology/Pain Clinic
University of Texas Health Science Center
5323 Harry Hines Boulevard
Dallas, Texas 75235
Attention: James Lipton, M.D.
Houston Headache Clinic
1213 Hermann Drive
Houston, Texas 77004
Attention: Ninan T. Mathew, M.D.
Telephone: (713) 528-1916

III: Attack Forms

Name _____   Date _____

                                  Day of week _____

                                  Time of onset _____

                                  Duration _____

Day of cycle _____ Days before next menstruation _____

During the 24 hours BEFORE the attack:

(1) Did you have any special worry, overwork, or shock?
(2) What had you done during the day?
    Normal work?   Unusual activity?   Extra tired?
(3) What food had you eaten and when?

Breakfast _____   Time _____

_____

Midmorning _____   Time _____

_____

Lunch _____   Time _____

_____

Midafternoon _____   Time _____

_____

Supper _____   Time _____

_____

Evening _____   Time _____

_____

Bedtime _____   Time _____

_____

What do you think caused this attack?

III: Attack Forms

Name _____   Date _____

Day of week _____

Time of onset _____

Duration _____

Day of cycle _____ Days before next menstruation _____

During the 24 hours BEFORE the attack:
(1) Did you have any special worry, overwork, or shock?
(2) What had you done during the day?
    Normal work?   Unusual activity?   Extra tired?
(3) What food had you eaten and when?

Breakfast _____   Time _____

_____

Midmorning _____   Time _____

_____

Lunch _____   Time _____

_____

Midafternoon _____   Time _____

_____

Supper _____   Time _____

_____

Evening _____   Time _____

_____

Bedtime _____   Time _____

_____

What do you think caused this attack?

III: Attack Forms

Name _____   Date _____

Day of week _____

Time of onset _____

Duration _____

Day of cycle _____ Days before next menstruation _____

During the 24 hours BEFORE the attack:
(1) Did you have any special worry, overwork, or shock?
(2) What had you done during the day?
    Normal work?   Unusual activity?   Extra tired?
(3) What food had you eaten and when?

Breakfast _____   Time _____

_____

Midmorning _____   Time _____

_____

Lunch _____   Time _____

_____

Midafternoon _____   Time _____

_____

Supper _____   Time _____

_____

Evening _____   Time _____

_____

Bedtime _____   Time _____

_____

What do you think caused this attack?

III: Attack Forms

Name _____ Date _____

Day of week _____

Time of onset _____

Duration _____

Day of cycle _____ Days before next menstruation _____

During the 24 hours BEFORE the attack:
(1) Did you have any special worry, overwork, or shock?
(2) What had you done during the day?
  Normal work?   Unusual activity?   Extra tired?
(3) What food had you eaten and when?

Breakfast _____ Time _____

_____

Midmorning _____ Time _____

_____

Lunch _____ Time _____

_____

Midafternoon _____ Time _____

_____

Supper _____ Time _____

_____

Evening _____ Time _____

_____

Bedtime _____ Time _____

_____

What do you think caused this attack?

III: Attack Forms

Name _____   Date _____

Day of week _____

Time of onset _____

Duration _____

Day of cycle _____ Days before next menstruation _____

During the 24 hours BEFORE the attack:
(1) Did you have any special worry, overwork, or shock?
(2) What had you done during the day?
    Normal work?   Unusual activity?   Extra tired?
(3) What food had you eaten and when?

Breakfast _____   Time _____

_____

Midmorning _____   Time _____

_____

Lunch _____   Time _____

_____

Midafternoon _____   Time _____

_____

Supper _____   Time _____

_____

Evening _____   Time _____

_____

Bedtime _____   Time _____

_____

What do you think caused this attack?

III: Attack Forms

Name _____   Date _____

                                    Day of week _____

                                    Time of onset _____

                                    Duration _____

Day of cycle _____ Days before next menstruation _____

During the 24 hours BEFORE the attack:
(1) Did you have any special worry, overwork, or shock?
(2) What had you done during the day?
      Normal work?   Unusual activity?   Extra tired?
(3) What food had you eaten and when?

Breakfast _____   Time _____
_____

Midmorning _____   Time _____
_____

Lunch _____   Time _____
_____

Midafternoon _____   Time _____
_____

Supper _____   Time _____
_____

Evening _____   Time _____
_____

Bedtime _____   Time _____
_____

What do you think caused this attack?

III: Attack Forms

Name _____   Date _____

                                 Day of week _____

                                 Time of onset _____

                                 Duration _____

Day of cycle _____ Days before next menstruation _____

During the 24 hours BEFORE the attack:
(1) Did you have any special worry, overwork, or shock?
(2) What had you done during the day?
    Normal work?   Unusual activity?   Extra tired?
(3) What food had you eaten and when?

Breakfast _____   Time _____

_____

Midmorning _____   Time _____

_____

Lunch _____   Time _____

_____

Midafternoon _____   Time _____

_____

Supper _____   Time _____

_____

Evening _____   Time _____

_____

Bedtime _____   Time _____

_____

What do you think caused this attack?

III: Attack Forms

Name _____ Date _____

Day of week _____

Time of onset _____

Duration _____

Day of cycle _____ Days before next menstruation _____

During the 24 hours BEFORE the attack:
(1) Did you have any special worry, overwork, or shock?
(2) What had you done during the day?
    Normal work?   Unusual activity?   Extra tired?
(3) What food had you eaten and when?

Breakfast _____ Time _____

_____

Midmorning _____ Time _____

_____

Lunch _____ Time _____

_____

Midafternoon _____ Time _____

_____

Supper _____ Time _____

_____

Evening _____ Time _____

_____

Bedtime _____ Time _____

_____

What do you think caused this attack?

III: Attack Forms

Name _____ Date _____

Day of week _____

Time of onset _____

Duration _____

Day of cycle _____ Days before next menstruation _____

During the 24 hours BEFORE the attack:
(1) Did you have any special worry, overwork, or shock?
(2) What had you done during the day?
    Normal work?   Unusual activity?   Extra tired?
(3) What food had you eaten and when?

Breakfast _____ Time _____

_____

Midmorning _____ Time _____

_____

Lunch _____ Time _____

_____

Midafternoon _____ Time _____

_____

Supper _____ Time _____

_____

Evening _____ Time _____

_____

Bedtime _____ Time _____

_____

What do you think caused this attack?

III: Attack Forms

Name _____ Date _____

                                Day of week _____

                                Time of onset _____

                                Duration _____

Day of cycle _____ Days before next menstruation _____

During the 24 hours BEFORE the attack:
(1) Did you have any special worry, overwork, or shock?
(2) What had you done during the day?
    Normal work?   Unusual activity?   Extra tired?
(3) What food had you eaten and when?

Breakfast _____ Time _____

_____

Midmorning _____ Time _____

_____

Lunch _____ Time _____

_____

Midafternoon _____ Time _____

_____

Supper _____ Time _____

_____

Evening _____ Time _____

_____

Bedtime _____ Time _____

_____

What do you think caused this attack?

III: Attack Forms

Name _____   Date _____

Day of week _____

Time of onset _____

Duration _____

Day of cycle _____ Days before next menstruation _____

During the 24 hours BEFORE the attack:
(1) Did you have any special worry, overwork, or shock?
(2) What had you done during the day?
    Normal work?   Unusual activity?   Extra tired?
(3) What food had you eaten and when?

Breakfast _____   Time _____

_____

Midmorning _____   Time _____

_____

Lunch _____   Time _____

_____

Midafternoon _____   Time _____

_____

Supper _____   Time _____

_____

Evening _____   Time _____

_____

Bedtime _____   Time _____

_____

What do you think caused this attack?

III: Attack Forms

Name _____   Date _____

                                  Day of week _____

                                  Time of onset _____

                                  Duration _____

Day of cycle _____ Days before next menstruation _____

During the 24 hours BEFORE the attack:
(1) Did you have any special worry, overwork, or shock?
(2) What had you done during the day?
    Normal work?   Unusual activity?   Extra tired?
(3) What food had you eaten and when?

Breakfast _____   Time _____
_____

Midmorning _____   Time _____
_____

Lunch _____   Time _____
_____

Midafternoon _____   Time _____
_____

Supper _____   Time _____
_____

Evening _____   Time _____
_____

Bedtime _____   Time _____
_____

What do you think caused this attack?

IV: Frequency Charts

	Jan.	Feb.	Mar.	Apr.	May	June
1						
2						
3						
4						
5						
6						
7						
8						
9						
10						
11						
12						
13						
14						
15						
16						
17						
18						
19						
20						
21						
22						
23						
24						
25						
26						
27						
28						
29						
30						
31						
Total						

July	Aug.	Sept.	Oct.	Nov.	Dec.

Name: _____

Year: _____

IV: Frequency Charts

	Jan.	Feb.	Mar.	Apr.	May	June
1						
2						
3						
4						
5						
6						
7						
8						
9						
10						
11						
12						
13						
14						
15						
16						
17						
18						
19						
20						
21						
22						
23						
24						
25						
26						
27						
28						
29						
30						
31						
Total						

July	Aug.	Sept.	Oct.	Nov.	Dec.

Name: _____

Year: _____

IV: Frequency Charts

	Jan.	Feb.	Mar.	Apr.	May	June
1						
2						
3						
4						
5						
6						
7						
8						
9						
10						
11						
12						
13						
14						
15						
16						
17						
18						
19						
20						
21						
22						
23						
24						
25						
26						
27						
28						
29						
30						
31						
Total						

July	Aug.	Sept.	Oct.	Nov.	Dec.

Name: _____

Year: _____

IV: Frequency Charts

	Jan.	Feb.	Mar.	Apr.	May	June
1						
2						
3						
4						
5						
6						
7						
8						
9						
10						
11						
12						
13						
14						
15						
16						
17						
18						
19						
20						
21						
22						
23						
24						
25						
26						
27						
28						
29						
30						
31						
Total						

July	Aug.	Sept.	Oct.	Nov.	Dec.

Name: _____

Year: _____

Bibliography

Abrahamson, E. M., M.D., and Pezet, A. W. *Body, Mind and Sugar*. New York: Holt, Rinehart & Winston, 1951.

"Amines & Migraine." *British Medical Journal* 693 (December 1967):23.

Arch. *Biochemistry* 85 (1959):487.

Blau, J. N., and Cumings, J. N. "Method of Precipitating & Preventing Some Migraine Attacks." *British Medical Journal* 2 (1966): 1,242.

Cochrane, Professor A. L., ed. *Background to Migraine—Third Migraine Symposium 24–25 April, 1969*. London: Wm. Heinemann Medical Books, Ltd., 1970.

Cugh, C. S. "Measurement of Histamine in California Wines." *Journal of Agricultural Food Chemistry* 19 (1971):241–44.

Cumings, J. N., ed. *Background to Migraine*. London: Wm. Heinemann Medical Books, Ltd., 1973.

Dalessio, D. J., M.D. "Dietary Migraine." *American Family Physician* 6 (December 5, 1972):60.

Dalton, Katharina, M.D. "Do-it-Yourself." *Migraine News Letter*. London: British Migraine Association, April 1975.

———. The Menstrual Cycle. New York: Pantheon Books, Random House, 1970.

———. "Migraine in General Practice." *Journal of the Royal College of General Practitioners* 23 (1973):97.

———. "Migraine—A Personal View." *Proceedings of the Royal Society of Medicine* 66 No. 3 (March 1973):263–66.

———. *Once a Month*. Pomona, California: Hunter House, Inc., 1978.

————. *The Pre-Menstrual Syndrome*. London: Wm. Heinemann Medical Books, Ltd., 1964.

————. *Premenstrual Syndrome and Progesterone Therapy*. Chicago: Year Book, Inc., 1977.

————. "Progesterone Suppositories & Pessaries in Treatment of Menstrual Migraine." *Headache* 12 (1973):4, 151.

Davis, Adelle. *Let's Eat Right to Keep Fit*. New York: Harcourt, Brace and Co., Inc., 1954.

————. *Let's Get Well*. New York: Harcourt, Brace & World, Inc., 1965.

Davis, Francyne. *The Low Blood Sugar Cookbook*. New York: Grosset & Dunlap, Inc., 1973, and New York: Bantam Books, Inc., 1974.

Epstein, M. T.; Hockaday, J. M.; and Hockaday, T. D. R. Radcliffe Infirmary, Oxford. "Migraine and Reproductive Hormones Throughout the Menstrual Cycle." *The Lancet* (March 8, 1975).

Gerras, Charles, ed. *Natural Cooking—The Prevention Way*. Emmaus, Pa.: Rodale Press Inc., 1972.

Hanington, Edda, M.D. *Migraine*. Westport, Conn.: Technomik, Inc., 1974.

————. "Preliminary Report on Tyramine Headache." *British Medical Journal* 2 (1967):550–51.

Hockaday, J. M.; Williamson, D. H.; and Alberti, K. G. H. M. "Effects of Intravenous Glucose on Some Blood Metabolites and Hormones in Migrainous Subjects." *Background to Migraine*. Cumings, J. N., ed. London: Wm. Heinemann Medical Books Ltd., 1973.

Journal of the American Medical Association 188 (1964):1108.

Journal of the Institute of Brewers 77 (1971):446–50; 15 (1972):25–29; 78 (1972):322–26.

Kent, Howard. "Yoga Techniques—The Treatment of Migraine and High Tension Headache." *A Report on a Controlled Programme with Migraine Sufferers*. London: Yoga for Health Clubs, 1975.

Kinderlehrer, Jane. *The Art of Cooking with Love and Wheatgerm*. Emmaus, Pa.: Rodale Press Inc., 1977.

Kohler, Marianne. *The Secrets of Relaxation*. New York: Stein & Day Inc., 1970.

Luce, Gay Gaer. *Body Time*. London: Maurice Temple Smith Ltd., 1972.

Mackarness, Dr. R. *Eating Dangerously*. New York: Harcourt, Brace & World Inc., 1976.

Marquardt, P., and Werringloer, H. W. "Toxicity of Wines, Food Cosmet." *Toxicol* 3 (1965):803–10.

Migraine. London: Office of Health Economics, 1972.

"Migraine and Diet." *Nutritional Services Quarterly Review.* London: National Dairy Council, January 1975.

Migraine News. Journal of the Migraine Trust, 1975.

Moffet, A. M.; Swash, M.; and Scott, D. F. "Effect of Chocolate in Migraine, A Double-Blind Study," *Journal of Neurology, Neuro-Surgery and Psychiatry* 37 (1974):445–48.

———. "Effect of Tyramine in Migraine, A Double-Blind Study," *Journal of Neurology, Neuro-Surgery and Psychiatry* 35 (1972):496.

New York Times Natural Foods Cookbook. New York: Quadrangle Inc., 1971.

Pearce, J.; Ron, M. A.; and De Silva, K. L. "Further Studies of Carbohydrate Metabolism in Migraine." *Background to Migraine.* Cumings, J. N., ed. London: Wm. Heinemann Medical Books Ltd., 1973.

Prevention Magazine. Emmaus, Pa.: Rodale Press Inc.

Sander, M.; Youdin, M. B. H.; and Hanington, E. "A Phenylethylamine Oxidising Defect in Migraine." *Nature* 250 (1974):335.

Somerville, B. W. "The Role of Progesterone in Menstrual Migraine." *Neurology* 21 (1971):853.

Steincrohn, Peter J., M.D. *Low Blood Sugar.* Chicago: Henry Regnery Co. Inc., 1972.

Wheaton and Stewart. *Analytical Biochemistry* 12 (1965):585.

General Index

Menu and Recipe Index